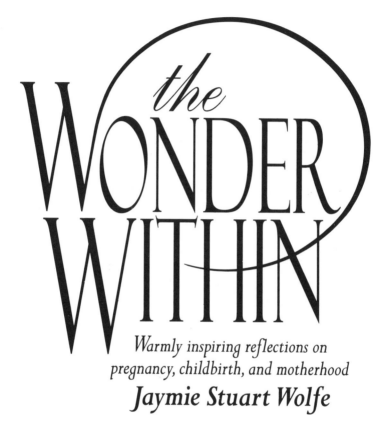

the WONDER WITHIN

Warmly inspiring reflections on pregnancy, childbirth, and motherhood

Jaymie Stuart Wolfe

AVE MARIA PRESS Notre Dame, Indiana 46556

Nihil Obstat: Rev. Romanus Cessario, O.P.

Imprimatur: Bernard Cardinal Law
                April 5, 1995

International Standard Book Number: 0-87793-558-0

Library of Congress Catalog Card Number: 95-78702

Cover and text design by Elizabeth J. French

Photography: David Hiebert 132; Rob Huntley 26, 58, 94, 118, 141, 166, 175, 186; R. Llewellyn/Superstock, cover; James L. Shaffer 82; Vernon Sigl 155; Justin Soleta 106; Sunrise/Trinity 52; Renaud Thomas 35, 161; Jim Whitmer 20, 41, 46, 67, 70, 76, 88, 100, 112, 127, 146, 181.

Printed and bound in the United States of America.

Dedication

To our holy mother, the Church,
who by the overshadowing of the Holy Spirit
births Christ in the world and nurtures him
in the hearts of her faithful.
As the handmaid of the Lord,
may she continually bear his fruit.

Acknowledgments

Writing a book is quite an undertaking. I could never have done it alone. First, I am indebted to my mother who, by her example, has shown me the way of loving self-sacrifice. Secondly, I am grateful for the undying support of my husband, Andrew. He is the most gracious husband and father I could ask for. It is he who has given me the gift of motherhood. Thirdly, to my five children I owe all my inspiration. It is for them—Jana, Nadja, Baby Paul, Kolbe, and Katerina—that this book is written. They are the jewels for which my life is the setting.

I am grateful also to my editor at Ave Maria Press, Bob Hamma. He welcomed my work from the outset, and has continued to treat it with the utmost gentleness and respect. His unfailing patience and insightful comments saw the project through to completion.

Lastly, I wish to thank the faithful priests that have made God's call to me both clear and irresistible. I am indebted to Bishop John Boles and Father John MacInnis of the Archdiocese of Boston, who cast the net that caught me into the fullness of faith, and especially, to my spiritual director, Father Paul Henry of the Archdiocese of Baltimore. More than he knows, he has been the midwife of a deeper faith in Jesus in my life.

May God repay them all with the richness of his blessings, for I never can.

JAYMIE STUART WOLFE, January 1, 1995
The Solemnity of Mary, Mother of God

Contents

Foreword

On April 24, 1994, Pope John Paul II beatified two Italian women. The new "blesseds" represent a whole class of Christian women whom the Pope refers to as "heroic mothers." The first is a woman of the last century, Elizabeth Canori Mora, who died in 1825 at the age of fifty. Her sanctity consisted principally in the maternal charity she showed to many families and children in need. This generosity was all the more remarkable in view of the fact that, a few years after their marriage, her husband abandoned her and their two small children. Blessed Elizabeth, sustained by a life of faith and the community of the Church, lived out her mission of motherhood with exemplary devotion.

The other woman belongs to the present century. She is Gianna Beretta Molla, an Italian pediatrician who displayed praiseworthy care for mothers, babies, the elderly, and the poor. However during her own fourth pregnancy, Blessed Gianna developed a fibroma in her uterus. The complications of this pathological condition threatened the safe delivery of her unborn child, but the doctor-mother instructed her physicians, "If you must decide between me and the child, do not hesitate: choose the child—I insist on it. Save the baby." Her daughter, Gianna Emanuela, was delivered safely, but despite the best

efforts to save both mother and child, Gianna Beretta
Molla died on April 28, 1962.

In his recent encyclical, *Evangelium vitae (The Gospel of
Life)*, the Holy Father explains why the example of these
two saintly women contains important lessons for the
world today. Noting the silent but effective and eloquent
witness that so many mothers give to the Church, the Pope
goes on to describe these women as "brave mothers who
devote themselves to their own families without reserve,
who suffer in giving birth to their children and who are
ready to make any effort, to face any sacrifice, in order to
pass on to them the best of themselves" (no. 86). Of course,
we are not surprised to hear these sentiments coming from
a Pope who, from the beginning of his pontificate, has
never ceased to insist on the importance of the family and
the special vocation that mothers and fathers enjoy in the
human family. On several occasions it has been my privilege personally to hear the Holy Father remind us that the
church considers each family "a Church in miniature." As
he further explains in *Familaris consortio (The Community of
Family)*, the domestic Church embodies "an intimate community of life and love at the service of the Church and of
society" (no. 50). We are all aware, at times sadly, how
much this service of the family needs to be strengthened in
our own nation.

In an extraordinarily perceptive way, Jaymie Stuart
Wolfe has seized the importance that Pope John Paul II
attaches to the family and the vocation of Christian motherhood. What makes her reflections on the life of Christian
faith so compelling is that she has developed them, as she
herself told me, "in the trenches." Now pregnant with her
sixth child, Mrs. Wolfe provides us with a personal account

of the high dignity of Christian motherhood. She invites us to share her intimate reflections on being pregnant, which she sets down with a warm and engaging style. At the same time, the author draws us into the everyday experience of pregnancy and child rearing. Mrs. Wolfe makes it clear that living out a lofty vocation does not exempt a Christian mother from sharing in the sufferings of Christ. No one will read this book without achieving a deeper appreciation of what the incarnation of the eternal Son means for the person who wants to live a life of holiness.

Although *The Wonder Within* chronicles the events that accompany a woman's pregnancy, it would be wrong to presume that this book will interest only women who are awaiting the birth of a child. Mrs. Wolfe provides an account of the life of faith that will enrich a diverse readership, comprised of all those who want to take up Pope John Paul II's challenge to enter into the service of the gospel of life. I especially encourage priests to make this book part of their formation for pastoral ministry. For it is important that we listen to the voice of a woman who has anticipated the Pope's call in *Evangelium vitae* "to promote a 'new feminism'" (no. 99).

The reader will not be surprised to discover that the Virgin Mother of God appears frequently in the pages of this book. Jaymie Wolfe has developed a genuine Marian meditation, one that will help all of us enter more deeply into Mary's faith. The author guides us along the path of Our Lady in a way that only a woman of faith could point out, and so illuminates the deeply religious significance that God has revealed in the motherhood of Mary. In *Evangelium vitae*, Our Holy Father again writes: "Mary is truly the Mother of God, the *Theotokos*, in whose motherhood the vocation of motherhood bestowed by God on every woman is raised to its highest level" (no. 103). *The Wonder Within* once again reminds us that every unity in the church is first realized in that of the mother and child.

As we approach the third millennium, the Holy Father has called us to a renewal of Christian values at every level of human society. I am pleased to commend this book to all persons of good will who want to associate themselves with promoting the gospel of life. In *Evangelium vitae*, Pope John Paul II reaffirms this strong conviction about the special vocation that women enjoy in rebuilding a world of human dignity: "Motherhood involves a special communion with the mystery of life, as it develops in the woman's womb. . . . This unique contact with the new human being developing within her gives rise to an attitude towards human beings, not only toward her own child, but every human being, which profoundly marks the woman's personality" (no. 99).

I thank Jaymie Stuart Wolfe for helping me to appreciate more fully the profound meaning of the Holy Father's words. It remains my special hope that many readers will avail themselves of the opportunity to listen to the testimony of a woman who in a real sense is writing for the twenty-first century.

> —BERNARD CARDINAL LAW
> Archbishop of Boston
> March 25, 1995 (Feast of the Annunciation)

Introduction

No matter how far our technology takes us or how many options we hold open, when it comes to the most important events or decisions of our lives, we have little information and even less control. We may think we have all the facts, we may use all the means available to exercise our influence, but in the end we are always left with the necessity of trusting the outcome. Sometimes we like to kid ourselves, and deny that we are trusting at all. Other times, we can feel frustrated when our lack of control becomes apparent, and the looming consequences of our choices overwhelm us. It is in these inner thunderstorms of insecurity and wonder that God calls us to himself.

For women, motherhood is probably the greatest unknown. A leap of faith here affects a woman for her entire lifetime — perhaps even beyond. For "traditional" women, the challenge lies in the apparently all-consuming demands of motherhood. We continue to struggle with issues of identity, and still often lack the support necessary to develop our own abilities in the context of mothering. For "modern" women, motherhood has become an even more complicated proposition. Our expectations are clouded by the sheer number of options we have. We are increasingly self-assured, but less sure of everything else. Our lives have all the grace of an elephant walking a tightrope. Convinced that we can have it all, we struggle to have it all at once. We are always rushing to catch up, and most of us never do. We are exhausted by the lives we have designed for ourselves.

In our explosive society of competing values, maternity itself has become a choice, and more and more a choice to swim against the stream. The intrinsic value of the uniquely feminine gift of bearing new life has not only been questioned, but in many ways supplanted, even assaulted. Consequently, the choices every woman makes are seen not just as her personal choices, but as the empty canvas on which she herself must define the very nature of what it means to be a woman. As the options for self-definition expand, that blank canvas can begin to look far more intimidating than inviting.

All of this is not to suggest that "traditional" women now or ever mothered in complete and organic joy, without fear, doubt, anxiety, or anger. Indeed, it could be argued that despite all our medical and social advances, and amid our barrage of choices, it is precisely these emotional currents that have remained constant. Most of us have at some time felt swept away by these emotional tides. Carried off into deep and unknown waters, many of us search for some compass by which to set a course, or at least find out where we are. But it seems that no matter where we turn for direction, there's something missing from feminine, or "feminist," dialogue.

Although for many, maternity is couched in the terms of whether or when, pregnancy and childbirth have remained a constant on the feminine horizon. We all know their transformative power in our physical and emotional lives. Yet few of us draw deeply enough to find what pregnancy and childbirth can teach us about our spiritual selves.

The expanding womb is not only the dwelling place of a life before birth, but a living invitation to expand one's heart for a Life which is in every way as dynamic and real as the unborn child. The child in utero is a living icon of the indwelling Spirit of God. Maternity is a parable of how we come to know God, and of how his divine life is manifested in our lives.

As our culture becomes increasingly pluralistic, we hear the debate between competing values grow louder. Both within the church and outside it, women are barraged by a continual stream of highly charged opinions about what womanhood is or ought to be. On the one hand, there are voices which call for ever more sexual liberation, abortion on demand, limited families, and the unconditional societal acceptance of lesbian relationships which, on their own, are sterile by nature. On the other hand, we experience a more "traditional" Church so unsure of what it ought to say about women that it rarely speaks to women. The result is that Christian women are generally left without a pattern of discipleship that is uniquely feminine. And the world is left the poorer, rarely hearing a spiritual voice that is both feminine and Christian.

Many of my fellow Catholics would quickly point to Mary, the Virgin Mother, as a feminine model of faith, and as the disciple par excellence. The truth of this is beyond debate, but as regards our own spiritual growth, what many of us have done with the Blessed Mother has not served us well. Instead of allowing her to lead by example, we have insisted on putting her on a pedestal so high that none could hope to follow in her steps. We have succeeded in abstracting her, and have torn her away from the emotional and spiritual constants of motherhood that all the rest of us experience. We clothe her in a garment of faith without doubt, trust without fear, and joy without anxiety, while we ourselves are wrapped in the rags of all those things, hoping always that no one will pull a thread hard enough to unravel us to the point where we become completely exposed.

Our Protestant brothers and sisters often do just the opposite, giving Mary little attention at all. Consequently, many view Mary as spiritually irrelevant to God's plan of salvation, if not functionally so. Some even question her faith and make her discipleship a point of contention. Her usefulness seems to vanish after the birth of Christ. Her motherhood lasts only the duration of her pregnancy.

Whether on a pedestal or disregarded, somehow Mary's own journey of faith is ignored. The only fruit of her pregnancy we seem willing to recognize is the child Jesus. But this is not the everyday experience of women who bear children. Each pregnancy bears not only a child, but a new dimension of spirit.

Because it is a journey towards new life, pregnancy is by nature a pilgrimage. It is not, however, a hermitage. The existence of the unborn child means that the pregnant woman is never truly alone — she is always "with child." Indeed pregnancy is not meant to be a time of seclusion, but rather a joyful sharing of what it means to be present, to be together.

Upon learning of Elizabeth's conceiving in old age, Luke tells us that Mary "went with haste to the hill country of Judea, to the house of Zechariah." In that visit lies the most compelling example of women sharing faith in all of scripture. The common feminine experience of maternity brings into focus for each the powerful life-giving Spirit of God. In Mary's journey through pregnancy as recorded in the scriptures, and in our own, we can, as she did, come to a deeper well of faith.

The Wonder Within is written in that spirit. Its purpose is to provide the reader the opportunity to see in pregnancy a model of spiritual growth. Through personal anecdotes and reflection, its intent is to create an experience of visitation, not just with the author, but with Mary, and ultimately with Jesus Christ.

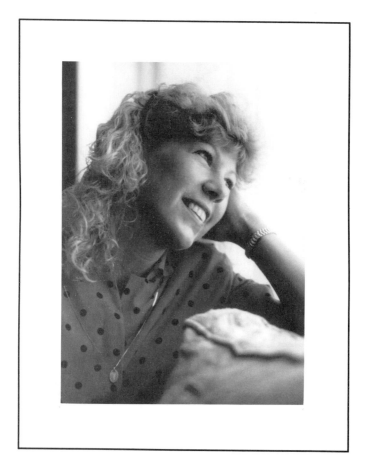

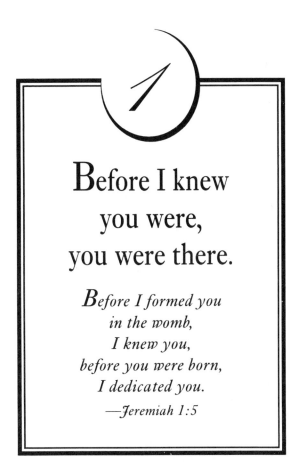

Before I knew
you were,
you were there.

Before I formed you
in the womb,
I knew you,
before you were born,
I dedicated you.
—*Jeremiah 1:5*

I'll never forget the first "annunciation" in my life. I certainly wasn't visited by an angel, but somehow, the experience of being made aware of a new life within me had that taste of awesome mystery nonetheless. I was twenty-two, married only six months, and living far away from any family. I had not yet had much time to make friends. I remember being embarrassed to take a home pregnancy test up to the drugstore cashier. I kept thinking that everyone was watching me, and wondering.

The little ring at the bottom of the test tube confirmed my suspicions. I felt startled and caught completely off-guard, just as if I had walked unexpectedly into a surprise party. I was at once thrilled and terrified, and wondered if this was all really happening to me.

Somehow, I just couldn't believe that I was going to be somebody's Mommy. I didn't feel pregnant, or look pregnant. The only evidence I had was that ring in the test tube, and the fact that I was a week late. Having a baby was something I wanted, but it was always a future proposition. All of a sudden, I had jumped into the future. The future was happening now.

A zillion questions flooded my thoughts. How did this happen (as if I didn't know!)? Would it be a boy, or a girl? Was the baby healthy? When was I due? Just how much was this going to hurt? What doctor should I go to? How was this all going to change my life? What were people, especially my family, going to say? The frosting on the cake was the frightening realization that I had absolutely no idea of how to care for a baby.

I felt tangled in contradictory emotions. Part of me wanted to go out and buy maternity clothes, to learn how to knit, to shout my news to everyone and anyone who'd listen. But there was also a place in me where fear resided, along with a desire to keep it all a secret, and a gnawing doubt that any of this was real.

We've all had the experience of being startled by someone who seems to appear suddenly from nowhere. Unaware of a person's presence, we go right along as if we're alone.

The person may be with us for quite awhile, but the instant we first notice her can really give us a jolt.

I remember having the sense at the beginning of each of my pregnancies that my unborn child had somehow crept up on me. I was dumbfounded at the thought that this new person had been silently growing inside me. It really is amazing that before any of us knows that we are pregnant, indeed before we even suspect it, the tiny life we carry within us is already there.

In the same way, sensing the divine finger tap us on the shoulder can startle and unsettle us. The very presence of God challenges our complacency, and reminds us that we are not in control. When we first experience God's presence, and know that he is there, we can feel disoriented — much as if we had awakened to find ourselves in a strange room after a long sleep.

It's reassuring to know that Mary had doubts and questions too. When the angel appeared, she must have wondered if she was seeing things. I always imagine her gasping at the sight and sound of him. The scriptures record him saying "Fear not," not because it sounded poetic, but because Mary was truly afraid. To be sure, if the angel's appearance was startling, no doubt his words to her were even more so.

In hearing his message that she would bear a son, Mary's first response is a quiet "amen." She asks the natural and immediate question, "How can this be?" The angel Gabriel is quick to tell her of the power of God, but adds the news of Elizabeth's pregnancy as well. Despite Elizabeth's barrenness and old age and Mary's virginity, the angel proclaims, "Nothing is impossible with God." Perhaps mystified, Mary gives her consent.

The scriptures tell us that Mary "set out and traveled to the hill country in haste to a town in Judah, where she entered the house of Zechariah and greeted Elizabeth" (Luke 1: 39). The journey was a long one, and doubtless took a few days. What a blend of excitement and anxiety she must have had in her heart. Like all of us at the beginning, Mary probably didn't feel pregnant. She had no symptoms, no medical test result, no proof of any kind, that what the angel told her was true, that is, if the angel really had appeared. She had to question if she had dreamed the whole thing — or worse yet, perhaps there was reason to doubt the source of what she saw. She had to go to see her cousin. She had to be sure. She had to know. Nonetheless, Mary abandoned herself to the meaning of the angel's words.

When Mary saw Elizabeth radiant and blooming at six months, she knew without a doubt the reality of her own pregnancy. Elizabeth testifies to Mary's maternity, saying "How does this happen to me, that the mother of my Lord should come to me?" (Luke 1: 43). How Elizabeth knew of Mary's child is kept secret from us. I'm sure the two women had much to talk about in those three months.

Like the presence of the child within the womb, the presence of God is not dependent on our awareness of him. We may not have any sense of his presence, any more than we do of an embryo growing within us, but God is with us all along. In the absence of any evidence, God is there. Before we are conscious of anything or anyone beyond our own existence, God is there. Even when we are wrapped up in the cloud of ourselves to the exclusion of all else, God is there. We may disregard God, we may think him irrelevant — even non-existent, we may not think of God at all;

but God is there, silently present with us, and growing to stretch and fill the space in our lives we allow him.

———————

Lord God, how wonderful it is that before I knew anything about you, you were there. You are everywhere around me, like the air I breathe — too small to be seen, and too big to be grasped.

Throughout my life, you have made your presence known to me in countless ways. Forgive me for the many times I've been so caught up in myself that I haven't even noticed you.

Awaken and startle me, Lord. Give my heart eyes and ears of faith. Let me see that you are never just "there," but always "here." Let me hear your voice as the silence beneath the noise. Help me to perceive your presence within me, and within all hearts who seek you.

Teach me how to be as present to you, as you are to me. and let my life announce your presence to all the world.

Amen.

———————

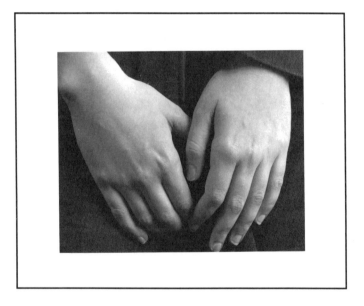

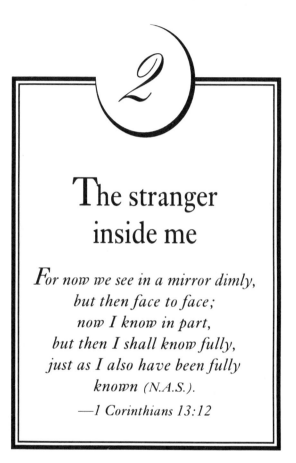

The stranger inside me

For now we see in a mirror dimly,
but then face to face;
now I know in part,
but then I shall know fully,
just as I also have been fully
known (N.A.S.).

—*1 Corinthians 13:12*

Most people would say that it's impossible to love someone that you don't even know. For myself, I've often wondered if it is even more impossible to love someone that you do know! I remember thinking about my unborn children as strangers, wondering about each of them, not only what they would look like, but what they would be like. I remember watching for their personalities to emerge as if I was waiting for the curtain to go up at a theater. I couldn't write the script. I was only the audience.

My oldest daughter was a real shock to my system. She loved dolls and tea parties and frilly dresses. She was naturally graceful, exhibited a full-blown maternal instinct from birth, and was adept at charming whatever she wanted out of unsuspecting adults. I remember her crying her eyes out at just over a year old because I hadn't done her hair the way she had wanted me to. She was, and is, the quintessential *femme fatale*. Sometimes I wondered where she had come from. She was so very different from me!

My second child, however, was in every way a chip off my block. Watching her was like looking into a timewarp mirror. She was assertive and direct, but extremely sensitive and big-hearted. She has a keen sense of fairness, is rather hot-tempered, and has a contagious laugh. When she walks into a room, she is noticed immediately. She just sparkles.

Nearly everyone we know has remarked to us about how very different our oldest two girls are. They really are like night and day, as distinct from each other as the breakfasts they eat — (one has dry toast and a grapefruit, while the other delights in Lucky Charms). Living with them and watching them become more of who they are each day has been an adventure.

Any mother of more than one child will attest to the fact that no baby is a "blank check." This became even more clear with the birth of our son. I had never really believed mothers who kept trumping up the differences between boys and girls. I felt all that was just an excuse for making "boys will be boys" — that is, "boyhood run wild" — the rule of the house. And boy, was I wrong!

The fact is that when we carry a baby, we are carrying an individual whom we choose to love regardless of who he or she is. Unlike when we marry, we have absolutely no control over the kind of people who will call us Mommy. Even with all our advanced medical testing, we cannot know what our children will be like, or even if we will like them. Many times I have marveled at the fact that if it were left completely up to me, I may not have chosen the people who are my own children as my friends! An even greater mystery is that somehow, despite their differences and ours, we manage to love them all.

Differences between children are evident even before birth. One child is quiet, another is active in the womb. One responds to music, another to a change in position. One stretches, and another kicks so hard that it's difficult to sleep. Newborns are unique too. My first child was content and serene, my second was a bit feisty, my third child was visibly observant, and my fourth very cuddly. One nursed well, another thrived on Similac after she refused to nurse at six weeks, the third threw up everything but soy, and the fourth was put on soy from the start.

Initially I had all kinds of expectations of what babies were supposed to be like. I was easily aggravated and annoyed by some of my children's character traits which grated against my own. But by the time I had our son, the way I thought about babies had changed. I became more patient, more understanding, more willing to bend to who they were, and much less demanding of who I wanted them to be. I began to see them as individuals caught, for a time, in babyhood. I no longer felt responsible to mold them, but rather to help them emerge and develop into the people God, and not I, had created them to be.

It finally began to dawn on me that God had placed these particular children in my life to help me emerge too. It really wasn't a one-way street. I have as much to gain *from* them as I have to give to them. Love challenges us not only to overlook what we may not like in another, but to rejoice in those things. Over the years I have learned to laugh at my own ways of doing things because, in all honesty, they make no more sense than do my children's ways of doing things. For better or worse (and that is up to us), we are all stuck with each other. They couldn't choose their Mommy, as I couldn't choose my children. But God has chosen us for each other.

We all like to think that we are the ones doing the choosing. But Jesus made it all very clear when he said to his disciples "It was not you who chose me, but I who chose you" (John 15:16). Mary and Jesus were chosen for each other. From all the women who ever lived, God chose Mary. God created Mary, not only to bear his Son, but to mother him.

Can you imagine knowing that the child you carried was the Son of God? What would he be like, what could he be like? Would he run and play like other children, or be some sort of a dreamy-eyed loner? What evidence would there be that he wasn't only human? But then, he was human after all, wasn't he? And how, oh how, would he grow up under her authority, the Promised One, the Anointed, the Chosen?

We all ask ourselves somewhere along the line if we are good enough to be mothers to our children. Mary, too, had to ask herself whether she'd be up to this; whether anyone could be. Could she go through with it? And as she wondered, the Divine Stranger, the Son of God and her son, secretly grew within her.

To God there are no strangers. God chooses to love us because we are his, not because he knows us, or *in spite* of knowing us. To us, God is the ever-present stranger. Like our unborn children God is always with us. And, like each child we bear, what we know about God is greatly outweighed by what we do not, even cannot, know. Nonetheless, God is intimate. He is at the very core of our hearts. There is nothing that stands between us; nothing that keeps us from each other. God is who God is — that is even his name. We cannot change God, or mold him, even though at times he may grate against us. We can only help God to emerge in our lives as he is.

Lord, although you are always with me, I hardly know you! You are closer than close, and yet very much a stranger to me. I've not yet even scratched the surface of all that you are; and yet, you know everything there is to know about me.

Sometimes you frighten me, Lord, because you are too great and powerful. And sometimes, you frighten me because you are too small and weak. I know that I have tried to mold and change you — instead of allowing you to mold and change me. I have wanted to make you more comfortable to be with.

Teach me, Lord, to embrace the mystery that you are — both the magnificence and the meekness. Help me to give you enough of my heart for you to emerge in my life in freedom and in fullness.

Amen.

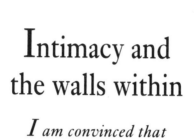

Intimacy and the walls within

*I am convinced that
neither death, nor life,
nor angels, nor principalities,
nor present things,
nor future things,
nor powers, nor height,
nor depth, nor any other creature
will be able to separate us
from the love of God,
in Christ Jesus.*

—Romans 8:38–39

It's funny how someone can all at once seem present and distant. In my own life I know that being there doesn't necessarily mean *being there*. Sometimes my thoughts, anxieties, or preoccupations have led me out of wherever I am and away from whomever I'm with, to a dreamy place where nothing can reach me. Whatever is happening continues in my apparent presence, when in all truth, I'm a million miles away, absent from everything that's around me.

When I have been pregnant, all that dreaminess seems to intensify. On the one hand, I'm absorbed by the reality of a new life within, constantly making plans and thinking things through. But on the other hand, all those thoughts and plans seem to focus more on myself than on the child; as if he or she was coming, but had not yet truly come.

The child growing inside me always seemed so very far away. Closer than close, not only *with* me but *within* me, I still sometimes felt as if this child belonged to someone else. At the same time I knew that there was no distance between me and my unborn baby. There was nothing to separate; nothing to keep the two of us apart. The very nature of pregnancy made us completely present to each other, and intimately so. To be sure, the wall of the womb is a thin one. The walls of the heart, however, are another story.

I had never had difficulty bonding with my first two children. From the moment I knew of their existence, I experienced deep feelings for them. My third pregnancy was much the same. I quickly invested all my maternal emotional stock into my new baby. But the pregnancy ended in miscarriage. I really wanted another child, and when I became pregnant again six months later, I was

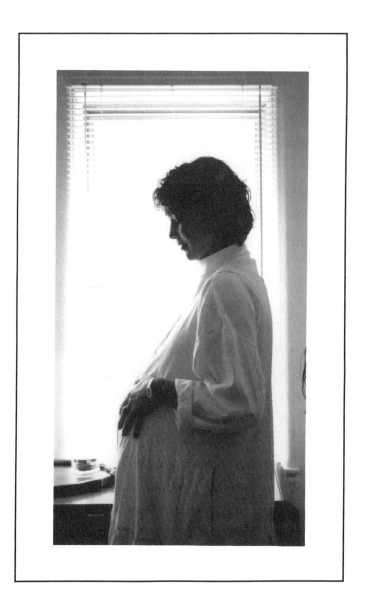

elated. Nonetheless, I found myself consciously refusing to become emotionally attached to our son before I had reached the third month of pregnancy. I held back my deepest love towards him at the start, because I still felt the loss of my miscarriage.

Instead of intimacy, I chose to allow my fear of losing another child to prompt my emotional defenses. I treated his very existence as tentative. I did not open my whole heart to him until I felt secure. In so doing, I failed to treat him as a person. Rather, I saw him as something that was *mine* — something that I could lose.

Although there are no physical barriers to intimacy during pregnancy, emotional and spiritual walls can and do create distance between mothers and their unborn children. These interior walls can be almost anything. Fear, stress, ambivalence, hurt, and even joy — can get in the way of our treating our unborn babies as persons, rather than as burdens or playthings. There is rarely a problem making enough room in our bodies for a new baby, but making room in our hearts and in our lives requires more of us.

Intimacy depends on each person treating the other *as a person*. We cannot be intimate with things. Similarly, we cannot be intimate with a thought, or a wish, or a *potential* person. Intimacy, wherever it exists, exists between persons. It is precisely the sharing of our humanity that makes the bonds of deep love possible.

When the Angel Gabriel asked Mary to bear the Son of God, he was asking her not only to share her humanity with her child as all mothers must, but to give humanity to God himself. When the Word became flesh, it was her flesh he took to do so. In order to dwell among us, he first had to

dwell within her. To come unto his own, he first beca
her own.

God's intimacy with us began with the intimacy he had
with Mary. There were no interior walls in her heart to
keep him at a distance. He was never far from her, because
she was present to him. As Mary so freely shared her
humanity with God, God freely shared his divinity with
her. God took up residence in her womb in the same way
that he had already taken up residence in her heart.

Through Mary, God acquired the humanity he shares
with us, so that he might become intimate with us. God
asks us to allow him beyond the walls within our hearts
that keep him far from us, even though he dwells within
us. God is simultaneously light-years away, and closer to
us than the air we breathe. He has no interior walls to keep
us from his heart. And because God is not an idea, a thing,
or a wish — because God is a person — the intimacy God
has chosen with us is possible, as we choose it with him.

...ny God, there is nothing that can separate me ...om your love. You assure me that all I have to do to find you, is to seek you. You tell me that if I listen, I will hear you knocking. You promise that if I open my heart to you, you will indeed come in.

But Lord, I often keep you at a distance. I give you part of myself, but not all. I draw lines in the sand of my soul, and tell you not to cross them. And when you offer me more, I tell you that I would rather have less. I keep you in a box large enough to hold closely what I desire of you, but small enough to prevent you from getting too close to what you desire of me.

Tear down the walls in my heart that limit your love. Teach me to surrender not only what I want to give, but what you long to receive. Show me that you do not approach to destroy me — but to embrace me. Help me to know that because you are Love, you seek me out; that because you lust for union, you pursue me.

Amen.

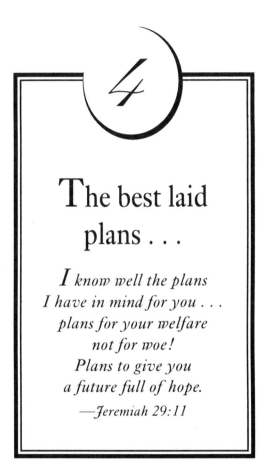

The best laid plans . . .

I know well the plans
I have in mind for you . . .
plans for your welfare
not for woe!
Plans to give you
a future full of hope.
—*Jeremiah 29:11*

Our world applauds both the desire and the ability to control our destinies. We are taught to emulate those who know what they want and get what they want, by treating life more as an investment portfolio than as a gift. I have fit quite comfortably into that mold. I have always had high goals, and have been successful in reaching them in large part because I orchestrate my efforts effectively. I have seen others, far more able than myself, fail to achieve what they set out to do because they did not plan well, or were unable to stick to a plan they had made.

Babies have a way of interfering with plans. Of our four children, three were not "planned," at least not by us. The first one came too quickly after we were married, and the second, too quickly after the first. The four years after that were a constant battleground between my husband and myself over whether or not to have a third child. He wanted more, and I was happy with the way things were. After putting up a good fight, I warmed up to the idea, only to miscarry. Finally our son was born. Our next child was right on his heels. They are seventeen months apart.

I know that when I'm not expecting to be expecting, and suddenly find myself pregnant, my whole world is thrown for a loop. It seems that just when I'm ready to move on with my life, I get pregnant. I have cried lots of tears over these "interruptions." But in retrospect, I laugh when I think that literally every time I have called for an application to a graduate school — law, liberal arts, fine arts, or seminary — I have another baby. (I have stopped making such phone calls!)

After two children in quick succession, I became convinced that if any of us were going to get what we wanted out of life, we needed to take control of this reproduction thing. At that time in our lives we used contraceptives to avoid another pregnancy until further notice. When my husband finally won me over to having another baby, we dropped the contraceptives and started "trying."

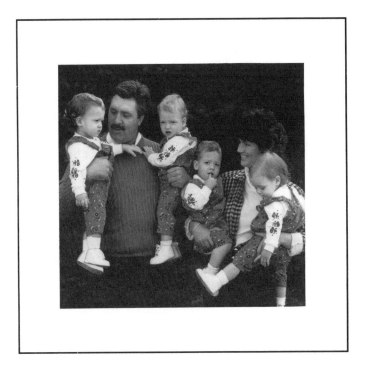

Once the decision was made, having a third child seemed a simple proposition. It had been all-too-easy to conceive before, so I was sure that all I had to do was throw caution to the winds. Two months later, I was pregnant. Everything fell into place according to schedule — until I miscarried. What a shock it was to discover that despite my planning, I was not in control. I had about as much success trying to have a baby as I'd had trying to avoid one.

I had been so sure that planning our family would keep things from getting too complicated; that it would free us from all sorts of undesirable circumstances. But I had never considered what I'd do if our plans failed. The strange thing is that somewhere along the way I had lost the very freedom that I was trying to gain. I had become a slave to the plans that I myself had made. I had fallen into believing that we were the only ones actively involved in our reproductive lives. I was wrong.

Our God is a God of creativity and initiative. Whether or not we have planned to have a child at a particular time, God has plans for us and for our children. The difficulty comes when our plans conflict with God's. Many of us talk about embracing God's will. But when it comes to the big areas of our lives, like childbearing, few of us trust God enough to allow *his* plans to take precedence over our own. Most of us spend our lives wrestling with the angel, instead of listening to his message.

Mary did not plan to become the mother of Christ. Certainly, it was not her ambition to be young and unexpectedly pregnant. Yet, even before the moment sin entered the world through the human heart, God planned Salvation to enter it through a virgin's womb. Jesus was God's plan — not hers, and not ours.

I'm sure if Mary had studied God's plan, it would have appeared ill-conceived. Under the law of Moses, the penalty for breaking a marriage betrothal and becoming pregnant with another man's child was death. From a merely human point of view, the wisdom of sending the Messiah in this way was questionable at best.

But Mary didn't evaluate God's plan: she didn't argue with it, nor did she seek to alter it in any way. The details, frightening as they must have been, weren't important to her because she had no intention of judging the plan itself. Mary was not the kind of person to trust in any plan. She found God alone worthy of such trust. All Mary needed to know was that it was *God's* plan. That was enough for her.

Unfortunately, most of us do not trust God with our lives as Mary did. Wanting to be responsible, many of us willingly take upon ourselves the heavy burden of deciding if, when, and how many children we will bear. But while we seek to plan our families, we often forget that God is planning his eternal family too. We shut him out when we treat our lives like sole-proprietorships instead of joint-ventures.

But as we grow in faith, eventually trust must win out over reason, and obedience must conquer willfulness. I often marvel at how the life I now lead looks precious little like the one I had planned. When I look into the faces of my children, I know that if it had been up to me alone, some of them would probably never have been born. I thank God that he has taken initiative in my life.

Whether or not you have a house or money in the bank, and whether or not you feel particularly ready to be a parent, there is no "good time" to have a child. There will always be sacrifices to make, and I think we kid ourselves when we claim that a "planned" child will necessarily be loved. Our children have taught me that "unplanned" doesn't have to mean unwanted or unloved.

It's easy to slip into thinking of new life, of children, as something *we* should and must plan. Yet, there is great freedom in realizing that there is someone else who is doing the planning. And there is joy in allowing him to do it without an argument. The freedom I thought would come with artificial contraception came only when we decided to abandon it permanently. Without it we leave the door open to *God's* initiative. As "in control" as I like to be, I am learning to give up trying to design my own life. I have yet to be disappointed, because no matter how good my plans are, God's are always better.

O great God of all creation, you have designed all the universe even to the smallest detail. You have placed each star and each blade of grass. From your hand comes every living thing; and not even a sparrow falls from flight without you knowing it. And Lord, you have designed each one of us for a purpose. You have plans not just for some, but for all, plans filled with hope and love.

But Lord, I have plans of my own. I spend all that you have given me to fulfill my wants and desires. Although I have asked you many times to help me set a course, I have rarely allowed you to take the wheel. I have often invited you along the paths that I have chosen, but have seldom asked you to do the choosing. I have sought your blessing, but not your will.

Lord, let my life's ambition be to please you. Help me to surrender my life into your hands. Set me, O God, like a precious stone in the place you have designed for me. And give me the grace to fulfill the purpose for which you created me to the glory of your name.

Amen.

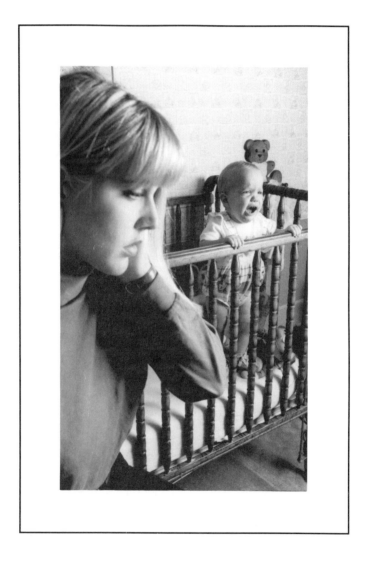

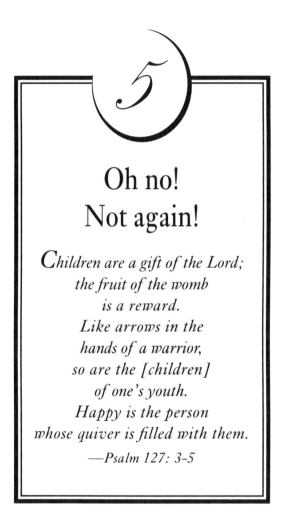

Oh no!
Not again!

Children are a gift of the Lord;
the fruit of the womb
is a reward.
Like arrows in the
hands of a warrior,
so are the [children]
of one's youth.
Happy is the person
whose quiver is filled with them.

—Psalm 127: 3-5

When I found out I was pregnant a second time, our first child was ten months old. I knew that I would want at least one other child, even though it seemed a bit early. But I wondered how in the world I was going to handle two babies. The best I could do was resign myself to coping with it. It frightened me to think that I was only twenty-three, and that I had a lot of childbearing years ahead of me. At this rate, I thought, I could single-handedly be responsible for overpopulating the North Shore of Boston, a distinction I wanted no part of.

To tell you the truth, the first six months after our second daughter's birth are a blur to me even now. I was absolutely overwhelmed, and found that it was as great an adjustment to have two children as it was to have the first one. The work wasn't that difficult, but learning to manage the relationship *between* them was.

I was so frazzled and inept at moving quickly between their needs that disasters just seemed to be a way of life. I remember putting the baby down to discover that my older daughter had exploited the irresistible opportunity to put an entire jar of Vaseline in her hair. Of course, it *had* to be the day we had an appointment with the pediatrician. So much for appearances!

I'm glad to say that things did get better — rather, I got better at holding everything together — if tenuously at times. I found that after the initial shock of having to split my attention and energies between children, they really did entertain and teach each other.

Nonetheless, I kept fighting the notion of having another baby. As I told my husband repeatedly, I was not about to be the vehicle for fulfilling what I called his "Abraham complex," that is his desire to be the father of many nations. I, for one, thought two was enough, enough was enough, and more was definitely too much.

When I stopped all that kicking and screaming, I found to my surprise that having our son was quite simple, hardly an interruption to our household at all. But when he was a mere eight months old, lightning struck again. All I could do was panic. My husband had lost his job three months before. The house we were in was too small. We already had three children in one bedroom, and our bedroom was being used as an erstwhile office for my husband's fledgling business. We didn't have the time, the space, or the money for yet another one. We didn't have medical insurance either. I kept wondering what in the world would happen to us.

The answer was nothing. We are still living in our too-small house; and there are still three children in that bedroom, (one child now bunks with my mother, who also lives with us). "Erstwhile" has not yet ended, because I'm still sharing my room with my husband's computers and file cabinets, as well as with my husband. And, we're slowly paying off the hospital bill.

Then again, something wonderful did happen. God added another beautiful child to our family. By the time she was born I had really hit a rhythm. Having her was essentially like Add-a-Kid. We named her after St. Catherine of Sienna, the youngest of twenty-five children. Just think how much poorer we all would be if her mother had stopped at twenty-four!

In watching our four children grow up together, I have come to realize that each of them contributes far more than he or she consumes. I find it hard to imagine our lives without any one of them. Because each one of them has something to offer, our whole family is enriched. Caring for them is not nearly so difficult as I anticipated. Larger families have a different dynamic than smaller ones. The older children help more than you'd think, and the younger ones don't stay young for long.

In almost every culture, large families have always been counted a blessing. But oh, how times have changed! In a world that shouts to us continually that bigger is better, and that there's no such thing as too much of a good thing, suddenly, it seems that when it comes to having children, the message of "more" no longer to applies. To venture beyond two or three children today is to swim against our cultural current.

I have to admit that I broke out into a cold sweat when my oldest child dedicated a story she had written in school to the hope that she would become the eldest of ten. But recently, I have come to terms with the possibility that I may not end up with just the four children I have now. I have resisted looking at myself as a mother-of-four, and have accepted that I may very possibly become a mother-of-more. (After all, God commanded Adam and Eve to *multiply*, not merely to add!)

The wonder of God is that he never stops creating. God is a master of multiplication. He does it not only in Bible stories like that of the loaves and fishes, but in our lives as well. God is always doing something new. God is always planting a new blessing, a new life, a new gift in our souls. Divine life is always fertile.

Few of us would ever want God to stop bringing forth new fruits in our lives. But somehow, we always seem to want to put an end to our own fertility, both physically and spiritually. We rejoice in our first few experiences of Christ's life in us, but somewhere along the line, we start wishing he would stop using us. We tell him in a hundred ways that enough is enough, that more is too much. We wish he would choose somebody else.

The Christian life of faith is a life always expectant. Indeed, the family of faith, the church, is not exclusive or limited, but welcoming and expansive. We all know that no matter how crowded it is, we can somehow make room for one more at the dinner table. Likewise, God asks us to persevere in joy, to expand our hearts, and to open our lives to *all* the life he wishes to give not only to us, but through us. God invites us to look beyond our own struggles and see *each* child, *each* fruit of discipleship, as a unique gift from him.

―――――――――

O Lord, from the beginning your love overflowed into creation, and from nothingness you called all things into being. The universe is filled with your works. There is no one who could number them.

But as wonderful as your creation is, sometimes I wish you would stop creating. Instead of allowing you a free hand in my life, I have often fought to hold you back. I have struggled to withhold myself from you, saying, "Enough is enough! I've done my share."

Lord, keep me in wonder at all you have made. Teach me to see all life as the unfolding of your creative and dynamic love. I give myself to you as an empty canvas to the master. Work your ways, O God, in the medium of my heart. Bring forth from my life all the fruit you desire. And at your pleasure, create and recreate me in your love.

Amen.

―――――――――

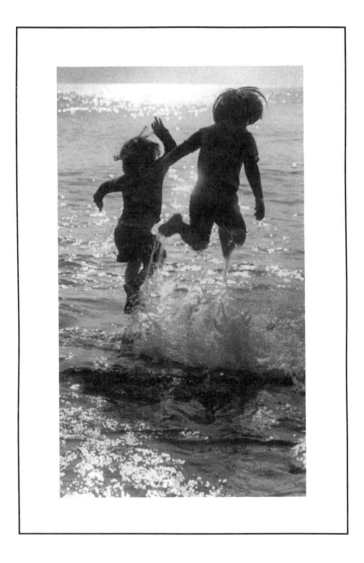

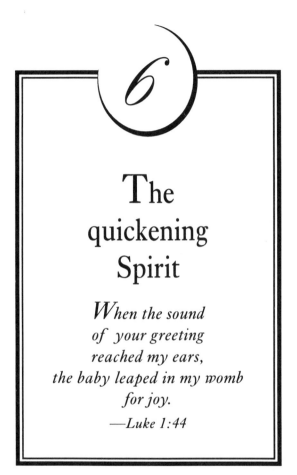

The quickening Spirit

*When the sound
of your greeting
reached my ears,
the baby leaped in my womb
for joy.*
—Luke 1:44

Among the blessings of creation, I believe that there can be no greater pleasure than the sheer delight of feeling new life stir inside us. With each of my pregnancies I could hardly wait to feel the movements of my tiny stranger. I remember eagerly anticipating that small kick to catch my attention, especially when I was expecting for the first time.

One day during my first pregnancy, when I thought that all my morning sickness had finally come to an end, I suddenly felt a flutter, ever so slight, of what I supposed was indigestion. I recall going to the cupboard to get out the Coke syrup, fearing that nausea would ensue; but it never did. The next day, I felt that strange little quiver in my stomach again. About a week went by, and I noticed that the flutter had become more frequent, and a little stronger. It finally dawned on me that my "indigestion" was really my baby. Oops!

The movements became more insistent every day. The flutters became tickles; the tickles became thumps; the thumps became kicks. Finally, by the seventh month or so, I could actually *see* my baby move. I remember how startling it was to notice that my dress was jumping while I was talking with someone. It was almost as if my tiny child had something to add to the conversation!

With my more recent pregnancies the rest of the family was quick to join in the fun. My older children even invented a kind of game with their new brother or sister. They would knock and poke from the outside, and the baby would answer in turn with a kick from the inside. My husband, on the other hand, preferred a more sophisticated approach. He shined a flashlight on my stomach to elicit a response. The strange thing was, it worked!

Years ago, it was thought that the first flutters in the womb signified that the child had "quickened," or suddenly come to life. Now we know that new life begins at the moment of conception, and that even before we can discern it, our tiny children are on the move. I sometimes feel sad when I think that even in successive pregnancies, my recognition of my baby's first movements was very much after the fact. Only when the quivers became kicks did I realize that those first sensations were from my unborn child.

Most of us relish the wonder of such movements, playing in turn by answering a kick with a pat. It's amazing that long before we can see or touch our babies, let alone communicate with them in any way, both mother and child engage in a mysterious and unspoken dialogue of movement, with a vocabulary of twitches, kicks, and turns. The gift of pregnancy provides us with a living dance of maternal and fetal love.

These movements, when we become aware of them, dispel immediately any lingering doubts we may have about the reality that we are indeed carrying a new life within. Every kick thrusts our unborn children further into our lives. Each stirring serves as a constant reminder that there is a hidden life inside us that not only exists, but moves and grows.

The quickening movements of God in our lives are very much the same. Like the first tiny stirrings of our unborn children, we often don't know enough, or are too preoccupied, to notice the movements of the Spirit. But noticed or not, the living Spirit of God moves in our hearts. God's presence is neither figurative nor still. God is a Living Being who is truly with us; who moves and grows in us like any other living being. His Spirit does not move in our hearts in grand and sweeping strokes at first, but the Spirit *does* move.

God moves in our lives in a hundred thousand ways. Sometimes the Holy Spirit flutters the gentle reassurance of God's presence; and other times, he seems to kick so hard that it hurts. He moves in both friends and adversaries. He prods and pokes at our hearts in both peace and in crisis. He moves in happiness and in sorrow alike.

When it comes to the things of God, we all seem to expect everything to be on a scale larger-than-life. We think that we will feel him in thunder and power, and strength, and so we often miss the signs of his life within us because they are quiet, and small, and weak. Eventually, as we grow in faith, we learn to recognize these movements as the Lord's. The quiverings of the Holy Spirit, however insignificant they may seem at the start, quicken in us the life of grace; and that *always* causes quite a stir!

The flutters, and pokes, and kicks of the Lord were nothing new to Mary. She had felt his Spirit move in her heart, long before she felt his tiny body move in her womb. His life had quickened in her so powerfully, that God made her the vessel through which he would quicken all hearts.

As Mary felt this child of heaven, this Son of God, dance inside her, what unspeakable joy was hers! That same joy can be ours as well. For like Mary, we can carry within us not simply a new human life, but life, divine life, eternal life itself.

Lord, it amazes me to think that you live so secretly in my heart, that you remain hidden and mysterious even though you are within me.

Overwhelmed by the concerns of my own life, Lord, sometimes I don't even notice that your life is moving in my heart. Lulled by the rhythms of my earthly existence, I fail to sense your dancing in my soul. But there are also times, Lord, when I think you kick too hard, times when your touch makes me uneasy.

Help me, Lord, to move with you. Stir up new life in my heart, O God, and quicken in me the fullness of your grace. Teach me to know your movements, however slight; and to accept them, however grand, that I may follow your every step with joy.

Amen.

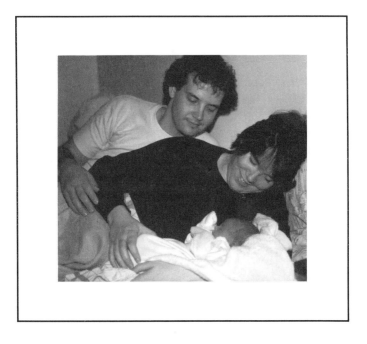

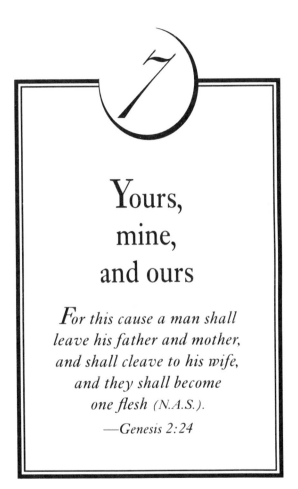

Yours, mine, and ours

For this cause a man shall leave his father and mother, and shall cleave to his wife, and they shall become one flesh (N.A.S.).

—*Genesis 2:24*

The ability to bring forth life lies at the heart of all that is uniquely feminine. No matter how involved a man is in pregnancy, childbirth, or parenting, he can never know what it's really like to bear a child. No man has ever had morning sickness, or has had to waddle instead of walk.

They may be expert Lamaze coaches, they may even be obstetricians, but men will never fully understand what labor and delivery feel like. On the other hand, a man can never feel life stir within him. And just as he cannot know the pain of birth, neither can he know the joy — a joy so deep that it overshadows pain. What a privilege it is to be a woman!

For me, maternity has been an all-absorbing experience. While my husband has remained well outside the world of the womb, I have been utterly consumed by pregnancy. That's why I have found it quite tempting to think of my children as only mine, especially before they are born. After all, *I'm* the one who's pregnant; *I'm* the one who's doing all the work.

My husband, on the other hand, seemed to me to treat pregnancy and childbirth as a spectator sport. Anyone who has ever seen a man at a baby shower knows what I mean when I say that he has always appeared very disconnected from the whole thing. He was never particularly attached to our children before they were born. He didn't spend much time speculating about gender, size, or temperament. His whole disposition was irritatingly hands-off.

I have desperately wanted my husband to be a part of it all. Recognizing his limitations, I have always made great efforts to include him in each pregnancy with endless updates and running "play-by -play" commentary. Invariably, I became frustrated with what I considered his lack of interest. No matter what I did, for him, pregnancy was nothing but a long wait.

I remember thinking one day how odd it was that my unborn child wasn't only mine; indeed, not even *mostly* mine. In truth, I wasn't just carrying *my* child. I was carrying a living part of my husband inside me too.

Even though I often acted as if it was just me and my baby, there was someone else involved in all this — unseen, and yet very much present. Somehow in the zeal of wanting him to share my experience — to be a part of it — I had failed to recognize that he was already very much a participant, and not at all a bystander. I began to see that although my husband could never know what it was like to be a mother, I could never know what it meant to be a father.

We often forget that our babies belong as much to their fathers as they do to us. No one would argue that maternity is limited to the physical. But many of us overlook the truth that fatherhood does not merely consist in supplying genetic material. There is a spiritual and emotional component of being a father, just as there is in being a mother. A man gives part of himself, the substance of his very nature, to a child. In truth, (and regardless of how they may act), our babies' fathers are by nature very much attached and not at all disconnected from their unborn children.

I am reminded of this connection every time I look into the faces of our four children. None of them resembles me much at all. Although I keep hoping that this will change as they grow older, they all look like my husband. My children's faces show me that my maternity is bound up with him. I would never be a mother if he were not a father.

No woman or man can bring forth new life alone. Children are a living fulfillment of God's plan for both men and women; that in marriage, the two shall become one flesh. They are the fruit of that marriage of spirit, and of mind, as well as of body. Each child is a perpetuation of that oneness, not just for a passionate instant, but for eternity.

There is a difference between seeing new life as a gift, and as a fruit. A gift is given by one and received by another. A fruit grows from a loving relationship so intimate, that it is unitive. Most of us are taught somewhere along the line that we should value life because it is a gift. But when Elizabeth cries out to Mary, "Most blessed are you among women, and blessed is the fruit of your womb"(Luke 1:42), we see that Jesus, the divine gift of the Father, is also the fruit of a loving and unitive relationship between God and humanity, between God and Mary.

Mary's maternity is cloaked in the fatherhood of God. The presence of Christ within her womb was a silent testimony to the presence of his divine Father. Jesus proceeded as fruit from the nature of each of them. From God came his divinity and from Mary his humanity. Heaven and earth are brought together in the person of Jesus Christ because his incarnation flowed from the meeting of heaven and earth.

The birth of Jesus teaches us that God does not act alone, not because he *can't*, but because he *won't*. If Jesus himself came into our world by the action of both God and Mary, we ought to know that his life within us depends both on God and on us. We cannot be his disciples any other way.

God takes the initiative when he gives us life in the womb, and when he gives us his life in faith and baptism. But we are not spectators in our spiritual lives. Although we cannot create the life of faith alone, it is not his plan that we be only receivers, but also co-creators with him.

Divine life, like human life, blossoms within us as the fruit of a loving and unitive relationship. If we make the mistake of thinking that we ourselves can produce such fruit, or that God will present it in our lives gift wrapped and without our participation, we will be sorely disappointed. Either we will become exhausted in the attempt, or unimpressed by the results.

But if we want the life of Christ to grow in our lives, like Mary, we must be overshadowed by the power of the Holy Spirit. Faith is a gift. But the *life of faith* is the fruit of our communion with God, in the context of our communion with one another. Our deepest hunger is for love, joy, peace, patience, kindness, goodness, faithfulness, gentleness, and self-control (Galatians 5:22). These fruits of his Spirit are not something we can achieve. They must be *fathered* by this Spirit in our hearts.

I thank you, Father, that you are at work in my life, that you are not a distant spectator, but alive and active in all I do. Lord, there is nothing I have, and nothing I am that doesn't come from you. Without you, Lord, there is nothing at all.

But sometimes, Father, I act as if my life is mine alone, and that even my faith comes from me. Trying to live my life for you, I often neglect to live it with you. Seeking to produce fruit on my own, I fail to seek the union with you from which all good fruit comes. And when I'm exhausted by it all , I wonder why you don't just give me perfect faith wrapped up with a bow.

Lord, keep me from becoming a spectator in my own inner life. When I want only to receive, show me how to give. Remind me that your shadow is brighter than my light. Overshadow my heart with your Holy Spirit, and conceive your fruit in my life. Protect what your right hand has planted in my soul, O God, and be the eternal Father of my faith.

Amen.

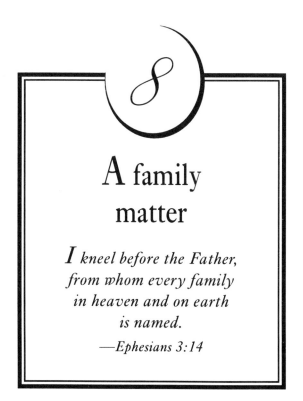

A family matter

I kneel before the Father, from whom every family in heaven and on earth is named.

—*Ephesians 3:14*

One weekend morning, as I lay in bed struggling to find the motivation to begin another day, our oldest daughter entered the room. She was six at the time, and very excited about expecting a new baby. She sat down on the bed and told me that she had been thinking, (usually a dangerous thing for most six-year-olds!) Then she came out with it. When the new baby came, she said calmly, she could kind of be its mother.

As cute as this notion was, I wasted no time informing her that I was not a surrogate for her or anyone else. I was the baby's mother. This was *my* baby. In fact, *every* baby that came into our house — past, present, and future — was mine!

As soon as those words left my lips, I knew how wrong they were. Of course my baby was mine, but not mine alone. Each child born to us was ours, but not only ours. Our children were not just sons or daughters. They were brothers, sisters, grandchildren, nieces, nephews, and more. All my little girl was trying to establish was that our new baby somehow belonged to her. She was right.

There is no greater joy than what we can experience as part of a loving family. In family we find our identity, and the security of belonging. We respond to the challenges that flow from our encounters with each other. We grow in love by yielding to one another. We rejoice in the sheer variety of life and faith, as we discover in others the talents we do not possess. Finally, we find the great satisfaction of working together as part of a living something greater than just ourselves.

No new baby enters the world in a vacuum. Every child brings with him a whole set of relationships. As our family has grown, I have become more and more aware that our children don't just belong to the two of us, but to our family as a whole. We are not only parents and children, but brothers and sisters as well. Each of us belongs to all the rest.

If Mary had ever made the mistake of thinking that Jesus was only her child, or only hers and God's, it couldn't have lasted long. Right from the start, the circle was ever expanding. Unless Joseph had been willing to

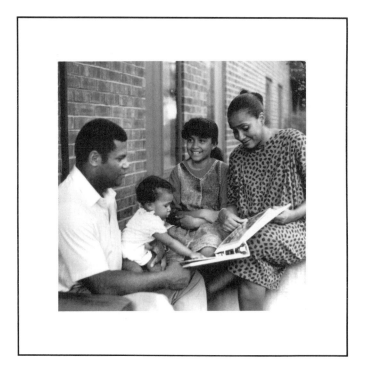

accept Mary's child as his own, Jesus may not even have
been born. Within hours of his birth, shepherds arrived at
the stable to claim him. Within days, Simeon prophesied
him to be the salvation of Israel. And within months,
Gentiles worshipped him as One belonging to all the
world. Jesus entered history as "the glory of his people,
Israel"(Luke 2:32) and as "a Light for the nations" (Isaiah
42:6).

The Christ we worship is both the Son of God, and the
Son of Mary. He is fully hers, and fully God's. But we worship Jesus because he is ours. He entered our world not
simply as the Son of God and of Mary, but as "the firstborn
among many brothers"(Romans 8:29). Each of us can claim
him as our own, because he came not just to establish the
Holy Family, but the eternal family of faith. Jesus brought
with him a web of intertwined relationships not just in
blood, but in Spirit. And just as in the flesh we are not born
sons or daughters only, so also in the Spirit, we are not only
God's children. In Christ we are brothers and sisters to one
another.

God places us and our lives of faith in families not just
because they are necessary or useful, but because they are
the ideal. Just as a family is more than the sum of its mem-
bers, the church is much more than the aggregate of
individuals sitting in pews. We become more than what we
are — more than what we could be alone — simply by
accepting one another as our own in the same way that we
accept Christ. Out of the unity and diversity that any family is, God makes us the Body of Christ.

Like any family, the church has its problems. We are not
always there for one another. We sometimes squabble over
how we think things ought to be done. We struggle to put

up with one another, let alone love each other. At times, we hurt each other deeply. But no matter how difficult family life can be, that is what the life of faith is.

Our claims to be the children of God are predicated on our belonging to the *family* of God. The measure of our belonging to him is as much the measure of our belonging to one another. If God is our Father, we will have many brothers and sisters. There are no only children in his household.

We cannot live the fullness of faith in a vacuum. Deep discipleship blossoms in a garden of many flowers. God gathers us to himself like an eternal bouquet. The beauty of a single blossom is not diminished by the crowd. But in its place, each one is enhanced by those around it.

Lord God, I thank you for calling me to yourself, and for making me your own. I praise you for being not only a Father to me, but a Brother, and a Spouse as well.

But, Lord, when I rejoice that you are mine, I often forget that there are others too. Sometimes I want to keep you all for myself, and pretend that you have called me, and me alone.

Lord, remind me that your arms embrace the world, and that in your eternal family there are no only children. Help me to accept all your children as my true brothers and sisters. Give me the grace to forgive those who have hurt me, and to ask the forgiveness of those whom I have hurt. Teach me to value your call in others' lives as well as in my own. And help me to glorify you in union with all who call you Father.

Amen.

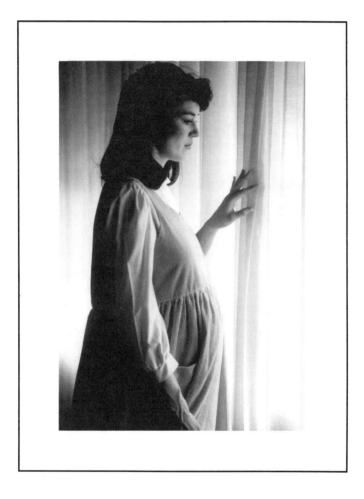

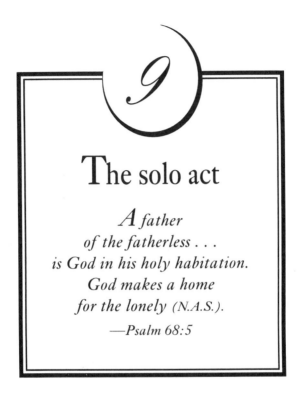

The solo act

*A father
of the fatherless . . .
is God in his holy habitation.
God makes a home
for the lonely (N.A.S.).*

—Psalm 68:5

Did you ever notice how just when you finally catch up with yourself, everything goes haywire all at once? Somehow, a strange and seemingly unrelated chain reaction of cause and effect erupts. There is a quiet moment, so the telephone rings. Just as you've finally found a comfortable position, and are almost asleep, you suddenly discover the urgent need to go to the bathroom. I'm convinced that the most effective way to wake a sleeping baby is to sit down with a cup of tea, and that the best way to ensure that your children go to the bathroom is to get them in the car! It's no wonder mothers are a bit paranoid.

In those frazzled times of utter exhaustion both during pregnancy and after the birth of my children, I have realized just how much I depend on my husband for support. Sometimes, when it has all seemed overwhelming, knowing that he was there cheer leading me on has made all the difference. And, even though I have yet to figure out a way for him to be pregnant *for* me, he has been pregnant *with* me. For while I've borne the brunt of carrying our unborn children, and then caring for them, in many ways he has carried and cared for me.

When I was pregnant with our son, the reality of my dependence, not only my husband, but on my entire family, became crystal clear. By the time I was four months along, my doctor alerted me to the possibility that I might be carrying twins. I was so huge by six months that people everywhere thought I was overdue. I remember going shopping and being amazed as the sea of people divided in front of me. It was as if they had seen a Moses standing in front of them, staff outstretched.

Any cause I might have had for thinking I was entirely self-sufficient vanished during that pregnancy. I was perpetually exhausted, had difficulty moving around at all, and was in constant pain. I had to rely on everyone around me: my husband, my mother, my neighbors and friends — even my preschool daughter. I often wondered what I'd do without them.

Unfortunately, more and more of us are having to find out what we'd do if we had to mother alone. How frightening it must be to embark on such a challenge — one that takes us to all our limits physically, emotionally, and spiritually — without the security of loving and intimate relationships.

Maternity was never meant to be a solo act. Just as it takes more than one person to bring forth new life, it takes more than one to sustain it. A woman is not created to mother her children alone, but with a man who fathers them. A man is created to father children in the context of a woman's maternity. He is always the father of her children, and she is always the mother of his.

Our fallen world is a far cry from God's intended ideal. Instead of families being a kind of symphony orchestra with each person playing his or her own part, many of us have wandered far from the score. We have ad-libbed to the point where the tune is barely recognizable. Forgetting our divine director, we have turned away from his music without ever having heard it, let alone played it.

Nonetheless, as Christians we ought to see in the eyes of every single mother a reflection of Mary. Often, we focus so much on Mary's holiness, that we fail to see her as those around her did. We want our Christmas images to be untainted by the notion that Mary herself was viewed as an unwed mother, and not universally acclaimed the Blessed Virgin Mother. Who would believe her story? I don't think I would have. Who *could* really believe it?

Mary trusted God not only with her body, but with her reputation, and with her life. When she consented to bear the Son of God, Mary had no guarantees. She knew that there would be no angel to answer the questions others would ask. She knew too, that not only would her marriage be in jeopardy, but her life would be as well. Trusting God may have begun to look rather easy when she realized that she'd have to trust her friends and family — and

Joseph — as well. What of all the talk, the rejection, the dishonor that was in store? Was this the "blessedness" the angel said would be hers?

But God did not abandon Mary to the law of Moses, her parents' disbelief, Joseph's doubts, or even to village gossip. Rather, God provided her with the support she needed not only to endure the circumstances of her pregnancy, but to rejoice in them. In giving his Son to the world, God did not keep his promise of salvation to all of us at Mary's expense.

Yet, unlike God, who does not turn away from the single mother, we often do. God saw to Mary's needs, not only the material, but those that were emotional and spiritual as well. God's call to the church is that we not abandon one another, but that we fulfill his law by bearing one another's burdens. Our single mothers are not virgin mothers, but God cares about them and for them as much as he did for the little Virgin of Nazareth. They do not carry the Son of God conceived by a miraculous union of earth and heaven, but all new life is miraculous, and all children are God's children nonetheless.

Lord, I thank you for all the people you have placed in my life — those who are there for me, and those for whom I am there. I praise you, God, for weaving us inextricably into each other's lives. You have shown us that it is love, and not weakness, that makes us dependent on one another and on you.

But Lord, when I am tired and have lost my strength, I often feel so alone. Sometimes it seems as if everyone has turned away. And at times, I wonder if even you have abandoned me.

Help me, Lord, to know the strength of your love surrounding me. Teach me that because you are with me, there is nothing I have to bear alone. Give me the grace to ask for help when I need it. And when someone asks for my help, give me a heart that will not turn away.

Amen.

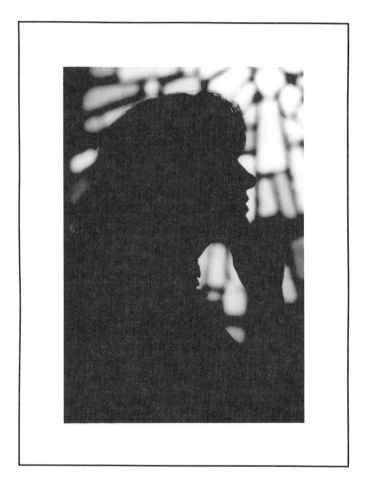

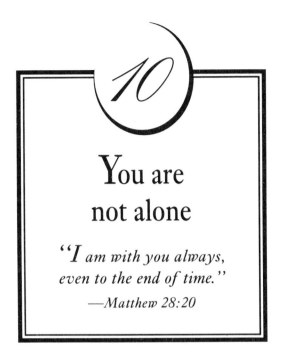

10

You are
not alone

"I am with you always,
even to the end of time."
—*Matthew 28:20*

"Pregnant" used to be an unwelcome word. Until not very long ago, our manners demanded that we use other, more delicate ways of conveying the news that someone was going to have a baby. We invented all kinds of euphemisms to keep our squeamishness about such matters intact. There were even ways of talking about "it" without having to say anything about her. Remember the stork, the pumpkin patch, and the doctor? So-and-so was never "pregnant," she was "expecting." (I remember as a little girl wondering just what she was expecting. I thought it might be something like a package from UPS!)

When we talk about pregnancy, many of us still prefer to choose from this more genteel menu of vocabulary. I find something uncomfortable in describing myself or someone else as "pregnant." It's not because pregnancy is scandalous in some way, but because the word itself falls far short of the depth of the experience. It is completely focused on the physiological alone. It is invasive when it comes to the physical details, yet evasive of the emotional and spiritual aspects of maternity.

Antique and out of fashion as it is, I think the best way of describing pregnancy is the phrase "with child." In reality, *presence* is what pregnancy is all about. No matter what she faces, from the moment of conception, a pregnant woman does not face it alone. She is constantly with someone else, physically, emotionally, and spiritually. The very nature of pregnancy requires a woman to be in the continual presence of the child (or children) she carries. She is always *with child*.

The pregnant woman is full, rather filled, with life — not just her own, but her child's as well. She is quietly occupied with the secret someone who is not only with her, but *within* her. Whether it be embracing or pushing away, she is abundant with interpersonal activity. Mother and child are alive to one another not only physically, but emotionally and spiritually as well.

At times this abundance overflows into bursts of energy. I remember stenciling a bedroom wall, cleaning absolutely everything, painting a few closets and bookcases, and even squeezing (and I mean squeezing!) between bushes to stain the front steps while pregnant. With much less fondness, I also recall fits of rage, uncontrollable tears, and emotional roller coasters that always seemed to be speeding down-hill.

Sadly, the spiritual abundance of pregnancy eludes many of us. Perhaps we focus too much on the physical realities that stare us in the face, and on the urgencies thrust upon us by emotional currents. We know in our hearts that there is something more, something *spiritual* to maternity. But somehow, it seems difficult to lay hold of that intimate spiritual significance for more than fleeting moments.

The sign that God would give to confirm the coming of the Messiah was that a virgin would conceive and bear a son; that his name would be called Emmanuel, God is with us. When the angel first appeared to Mary, his greeting to her might have seemed strange. It is the greeting we recall with familiarity when we pray the Hail Mary. In Mary's spirit the angel recognizes the fullness of the Holy Spirit. "Full of grace," he says; "the Lord is with you."

Mary, indeed, was full of grace. She blossomed like the flower for whom the entire garden was cultivated; like the plant that had never been outside the greenhouse of God's presence. She had been caught up into the divine love of the Trinity. The fullness of her grace flowed from that same divine love.

In some respects, becoming the mother of the Savior did not change Mary's relationship with God much at all. Even before her assent to the will of God, the angel had called her "full of grace." Even before she actually conceived, he had already told her "the Lord is with you."

When Mary was with child, she was in the physical presence of the Lord who had always been with her spiritually. She was with him continually, just as we are all continually with our unborn children. Can you imagine the God who created all the heavens and the earth being *with*, even *within* you?

The very wonderful thing is that through faith and baptism we no longer have to imagine. The presence of God is as real and as close as the presence of our children in the womb. We voice this hidden truth whenever we call God our Father. We see it in the scriptures that tell us that it is "in him we live, and move, and have our being" (Acts 17:28). God is the world in which our spirits live and grow.

We are filled with grace from the very same God who filled the heart of Mary. It is that grace which confines the awesome divine presence *within* our hearts and lives in the same way that Jesus was confined in the womb of Mary— and just as our children are held captive for a time within our bodies. It may have been enough for us to have God with us, but it was not enough for him. God's thirst for intimacy could not be quenched by simply being *with* — he had to be *within*.

God's greatest desire is that we be as present to him as he is to us, that we be not only with him, but within him, and that he be within us. Presence has always been the promise and the purpose of God's plan. There is not a moment of our lives when God is absent. God does not, will not, abandon us. We can live our lives with confidence, knowing that we are never truly alone. We are always with him, because he is Emmanuel — not only for Mary, but for us and all the world.

*L*ord, you have shown me that from the moment my life began, I have never been alone. Because I am part of the pulse of life, my whole being teems with the activity that surrounds me.

But although my life is lived in the continual presence of others, I often become preoccupied with myself. I rush along emotional currents too quickly to sense the significance of another's presence. I grasp onto my own experience, without understanding that the life that surrounds me — and the life that moves inside me — is not simply my own.

Lord, teach me to be attentive to others. Empty me of myself and fill me with your presence. Quench your thirst for intimacy with my soul. In the midst of all my frantic activity, give me peace. Make my heart your temple, and my life a place where all I meet encounter you.

Amen.

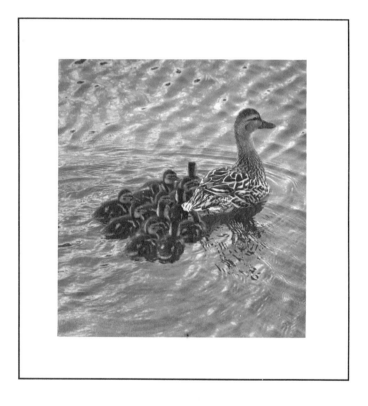

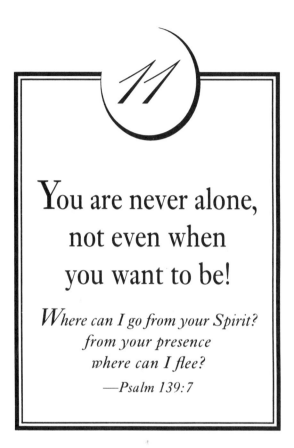

You are never alone, not even when you want to be!

Where can I go from your Spirit?
from your presence
where can I flee?

—*Psalm 139:7*

How comforting it is to know that we are never truly alone — and how aggravating it is when we want to be! I have found that there are limits to how long I can stand just being around people, even those I love. Many of us have witnessed the breakup of good friendships simply because of what I call "overdose." There does seem to be such a thing as being together too much.

A few years ago, my husband lost his job, and we decided that he would try building a business of his own. In the absence of other choices, he set up shop in a corner of our bedroom. Although he spent more and more hours isolated behind that bedroom door, I felt his continual presence cramping my style. Just knowing he was there began to grate on me. I kept wishing he would just *get out of my house!*

But if absence really does make the heart grow fonder, what of the woman who is inescapably with child? There is no way a pregnant woman can distance herself from her baby. There is nothing she can do to get some space. There are no boundaries that can be drawn between them. They are always together. They are never alone. And although the depth and joy of pregnancy is rooted in this intimacy, it is precisely this intimacy that can really begin to grate on our nerves.

Even before her baby is born a mother is on-call. Her body is at her child's disposal. A first-time mother learns quickly that maternity is more than a full-time job. The business of having a family is very much like a family business. It is a venture with convenience store hours — and it's not her convenience that comes first.

As wonderful as it is to be with child, there are times that all of us desperately want to be alone. Growing up as an only child, I think that I have been particularly sensitive to this loss of solitude, especially between the hours of eleven at night and seven in the morning! I have seen my children struggle with this too. As much as they love the new baby, they can really get tired of having to change their plans and patterns to accommodate her. Toddlers, they have discovered, are expert wrecking crew material.

Maternity pushes us to all our limits, and beyond. Not only our physical energy, but our emotional resources can be easily spent up. There is no human state that is more demanding or consuming. Sometimes I have imagined myself wearing an "Occupied" sign around my neck and I have often wondered how I might trade it in for a "Do Not Disturb!"

Our lives of faith are not unlike pregnancy in these respects. There are certainly times that I grow tired of feeling God breathe down the back of my neck; times when I wish that the "Hound of Heaven" would bark up some other tree. I am never quite sure how to respond. The strangeness, mystery, and novelty of the divine presence is undeniably attractive. But the intimacy God pursues is often annoying and unnerving.

Many of us spend our entire lifetimes caught in that dilemma. We run from what we perceive as the endless demands of God in our lives. We search everywhere for a place to hide. We throw up our hands when we find that there is none.

I can imagine Mary experiencing this. From the very little we know about her life, it may have seemed to Mary as if things would never be quiet again. As soon as one thing was resolved, three others took its place.

She consents to conceive the Son of God, only to find herself at a loss to explain it all to Joseph. An angel appears and Joseph's doubts disappear, but then they are required to travel to Bethlehem. When they arrive, there is no room for them — except in a cave. The baby is born, but the moments just after the birth are interrupted by a ragged band of shepherds, almost indistinguishable from their sheep, at least in terms of odor.

When the infant Jesus is presented at the Temple as pre-scribed by Jewish law, the prophet Simeon proclaims him to be the Savior. But his words to Mary about a sword that was to pierce her heart cast a shadow on the joy. Finally, just as everything seems to calm down, wise men arrive in Bethlehem. The good news is that they brought gifts; the bad news is that Herod wants to kill the child. They must flee to Egypt.

This whirlwind is what we celebrate as the "Joyful Mysteries." We often say that when it rains, it pours. Mary must have felt as if she were caught in the great flood!

Mary could have chosen to flee from God, just as she had fled from Herod's wrath. But instead Mary lived by faith. She could not abandon the One who would not aban-don her. Mary knew that God was more available to her than she could ever be to him. Instead of running away from his presence, she ran towards it. Instead of struggling against him, she conformed herself to him. She trusted that because there was no place to hide from God, that he would be her hiding place from all that makes life difficult.

I have come to the conclusion that shaking your fist at the inevitable is even more exhausting than accepting it. There is a certain interior peace that comes when — and only when — we surrender to the limitations of our lives. All the interruptions, the noise, the commotion, and even our own frustrations — these things are external to moth-ering. They do not have to contribute to an inner desperation.

Maternity is much deeper than that. A mother I am, and a mother I will be. It is not what I *do*; it is bound up in who I *am*.

When we are overwhelmed by the inescapable responsibilities of motherhood, we must remember that our children's very lives depend on our presence. Likewise, when we tire of God's presence in our lives, when we want him to leave us alone, we must recall that he has created us for the purpose of being with him not only for a moment, but for all eternity. We are attached to him forever by the umbilical cord of our faith and baptism. We are as dependent upon him as the unborn children we carry. To seek an escape from his presence, is to turn away from life itself.

Lord, as grateful as I am to have you near, I have to admit that there are times I wish you would leave me alone. At those times, O God, your invitations sound like demands, your breath feels like a whirlwind, and your touch irritates more than comforts.

I have tried all the escape routes I could find, but no matter where I've run or turned, you have always been there waiting. Afraid of what going deeper might mean, I have exhausted myself contending with you. My arms have grown weary from pushing you away.

Lord, help me to remember that without you there is nothing, and that beyond you there is only darkness. When I grow resentful of my dependence on you, teach me to be grateful for all you have done for me. When I try to run away, run after me, Lord. Catch me in your arms, and carry me into eternity with you.

Amen.

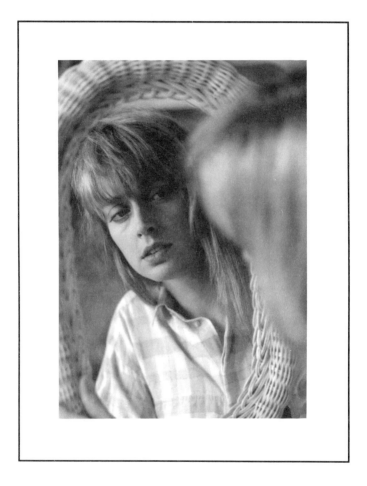

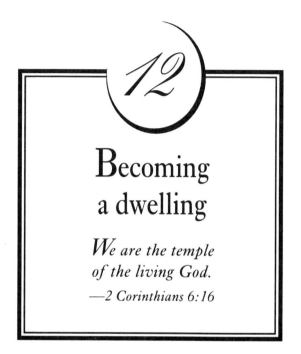

12

Becoming a dwelling

We are the temple of the living God.
—*2 Corinthians 6:16*

Most of us are intrigued by how we look when we're expecting. We all marvel at how our bodies change shape. We study our profiles in the mirror with both shock and delight. We ask our friends and mates about how much we "show." First-time mothers try to imagine just how far they'll have to sit from the dinner table at the end. Experienced mothers catch themselves making comparisons between pregnancies.

When I was carrying our second child, a few of our friends were expecting children as well. One morning after church, my husband observed that seeing us all together was much like being on a whale watch. Not all of us appreciated this remark. For myself, I enjoyed a good laugh out of it.

There is something undeniably funny about how we look when we're pregnant. The Einstein factor enters in here. Size is relative. Being only five foot two inches tall has put me at a disadvantage. The babies I carry have nowhere to grow but out. To make it worse, all four of our children were over nine pounds at birth — (our son was a whopping ten pounds fifteen ounces!). I have often joked about looking like a piece of real estate.

All joking aside, there is some truth to the notion that maternity doesn't just make us look like a house, it actually turns us into one. While we are pregnant, our bodies are our baby's home. We are where they live.

It is a warm and welcoming spirit that makes a house a home. Likewise, it is the same kind of warmth that transforms not only our bodies, but our lives into "home" for all our children. Fewer and fewer of us list our occupation as "homemaker." Yet, in a real sense, that is what every mother is called to be. The physical nature of maternity gives us no choice. Our unborn children inhabit our bodies whether we like it or not. But emotionally, and spiritually, *we* do the choosing. We all become houses; but we do not all become homes. Many of us do not prepare our hearts to receive our children as diligently as we might prepare our homes to receive a guest. We leave our lives cluttered and disordered. We fail to attend to the needs of our children. Sometimes, we even abandon them. We do not put ourselves at their disposal, or welcome them with all that we are.

The Lord who made the heavens and the earth, who all the universe cannot contain, chose to dwell in the womb of

Mary. When God came to her, he did not find her unprepared. Her heart was pure and open. Her soul was still. Her whole spirit was waiting to submit. Mary received the Divine Guest readily.

Similarly, when Mary goes to visit her cousin Elizabeth, she comes as a guest to her cousin's home. Elizabeth, honored by her presence, asks, "Who am I that the mother of my Lord should come to me?" Although she has plenty of needs herself, Elizabeth places herself at the disposal of her guest. In so doing, she welcomes into her life both Mary and the child she carries.

Mysteriously, even the unborn infant John welcomes Christ as a guest. He leaps for joy at the hidden presence of the divine child who makes his home in Mary. He dances before him as David danced before his presence in the Ark of the Covenant. In bearing the Son of God, Mary becomes the Ark of the *New* Covenant. She becomes the home of God's salvation.

Indeed, Mary was the first person who became the dwelling place of God's presence, but she was not the last. Throughout history, holy men and women have placed themselves completely at God's disposal. God wishes to make *each one of us* his home. He first took up residence in Mary's body, so that he could then reside in all our hearts.

The Gospel of John tells us that "The Word became flesh, and dwelt among us"—literally, that God "pitched his tent" with us. Through faith it is possible for each of us to become the tent he pitches, the place in which he dwells. To do so, we must learn to practice hospitality. We must receive God in the same way that Elizabeth received Mary. We must resist the temptation to feel put out. When he comes, we must greet him with the joy a host has at the arrival of a much longed-for guest. Our spirits must learn to dance before him.

It is much easier to receive a friend than it is to receive a stranger. Many of us claim to desire intimacy with God. But we can never expect to embrace him as a friend or brother or lover, unless we first learn to welcome him as a stranger. Whoever God becomes to us in our lives, he appears to us first as the Divine Stranger. He approaches us as One who is looking for a place to dwell. Our parents may well have taught us to beware of strangers. But the scriptures teach us "Do not neglect to show hospitality to strangers, for some have entertained angels without knowing it" (Hebrews 13: 2 N.A.S.).

Like our wombs that stretch to become dwelling places for our unborn children, our hearts — small as they are — can become home for God himself. We need not be grand and glorious country mansions. We need only prepare, and make room. Our lives are the poor stables in which he wants to be born; our hearts, the mangers in which he longs to rest; our souls, the castles in which he hopes to dwell.

O Lord, all the brilliance of creation is but a candle to the splendor of your presence. You shine more gloriously than the stars; you reach above the heights of heaven and you stand below the depths of the earth. You are so vast that not even the whole universe can contain you.

But it is not on high mountains, nor in ocean depths that you wish to dwell. You do not seek rich palaces to give you glory, but rather, human hearts.

Lord, give me a warm and welcoming spirit. Help me to always greet you with joy. Teach me to make room for you in preparation for your coming. Be born in the poor stable of my life, O God. Come, make your home in my heart.

Amen.

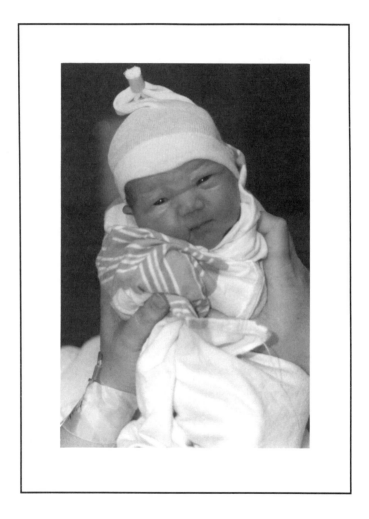

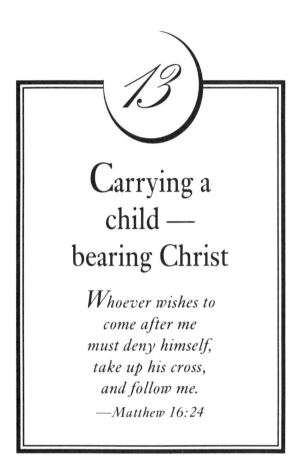

Carrying a child — bearing Christ

Whoever wishes to come after me must deny himself, take up his cross, and follow me.

—*Matthew 16:24*

There's nothing new or exotic about maternity. As long as there have been women, women have passed through pregnancy. All around the world, and for thousands of years, having babies has been the stuff of everyday human existence. Nonetheless, pregnancy continues to hold our attention. Whether we are men or women, first-time mothers, experienced mothers, or not mothers at all — we find the process of pregnancy and birth fascinating.

Somehow, childbirth is never old news. When it is happening to us or to someone we know, it feels new all over again. Like a rarely used spice hidden in the back of the cupboard, I would have expected maternity to lose some of its flavor. But to my surprise, I have found my wonder increase with each experience of it. Even after four children, for me, pregnancy is every bit as awesome as it was the first time.

Trying to explain maternity to our older children has heightened my own sense of the mystery of it all. I'll never forget the struck-by-lightning look on my preschooler's face when she finally grasped what I was telling her. When we were expecting the fifth time, my sophisticated third grader still showed the glimmer of an "I'm-not-sure-if-I-buy-this." The mix of joy and wonder they have expressed has most definitely contributed to my own.

The wonder of pregnancy, however, does not negate its challenges. Maternity is never a breeze, even if and when it feels like one. I felt great when I was expecting our first child. I was not going to treat pregnancy like an illness. I couldn't understand why pregnant women are always being told to "take care of themselves."

I recall feeling exasperated at times by some of the well-intentioned, but unsolicited advice people kept on giving me. Even strangers seemed to come out of the woodwork touting conventional wisdom. But, many of us ought to admit that we relish the extra attention and pampering we get while we're expecting. Some of us have developed it into quite a racket, at least at times!

The extra consideration we receive is offered because people recognize that pregnancy is in a certain sense burdensome. Those who notice that we are expecting respond to us in much the same way as they do when they see someone elderly board a crowded bus. Their kindnesses flow from the awareness that childbearing means *bearing* a child.

On a purely physical level, pregnancy requires us to put ourselves out. The child in the womb takes what he needs from our bodies, while we ourselves get only what's left over. Those gigantic vitamins are, in truth, more for us than they are for our babies. They are prescribed because maternity depletes us.

While we make the day to day sacrifices of maternity without a second thought, we fall out of touch with the very personal nature of those sacrifices. Many of us abstract from what we are doing, and forget why we are doing it. No one in her right mind would voluntarily feel sick, gain weight, or carry around a bowling ball for several months. The reason we put ourselves out in these and so many more ways is not found in a principle, or even in the process, but in a person.

We put our own lives on the back burner, not as an end in itself, but because that is what our children require. Our pregnancies are a nine-month-long baby shower in which we give our babies our bodies and our lives. We count it a joy not because we are so holy or magnanimous, but because we do it for love. That love is never indiscriminate or impersonal. It is given by a particular woman to a particular child.

Sometimes, I have found it difficult to remain focused on the fact that no one is generically pregnant. I mean that none of us carries a baby or "the baby," but rather a unique and individual person within us. The changes we experience often distract us from thinking in this way. We tend to lose our awareness of the fact that underneath all that belly is a *who*, and not a *what*.

For Mary, that who was the Son of God. The difficulties she faced were not exacted from her like some kind of payment to a divine creditor. The sacrifices she made were not part of some abstract spiritual exercise. What Mary bore was for love of *whom* Mary bore. She put her own desires and concerns on hold not because it was asked of her, but because *he* had asked it of her.

The Church proclaims Mary the *Theotokos*, or God-bearer. Through her, God entered humanity. But Mary not only brought Christ into the world; she was also his disciple. Her total gift of herself to God is a mirror of God's sacrificial gift to us. Because he loved us, Jesus bore us and our sins when he carried the cross. But long before Jesus carried the cross, Mary carried him.

We bear within our hearts not someone unknown to us, but that very same Christ. We are the objects of his love, a love which is no less personal than our own. This passionate love for us made his great sacrifice both meaningful and possible. Through it, Jesus not only carried a cross up a hill, but bore us and all we are up to heaven. He gave his life not only for us, but to us. It is that kind of loving sacrifice and self-denial that God invites us to embrace.

O Lord, our lives are filled with joy and wonder. Even in the most mundane and ordinary things, you are always giving us something new. You bury rich treasures in the rhythms of our days. You are forever showing us that there is so much more to life than what we can see.

But Lord, I rarely bask in the wonder of your creation. My soul is drained with exhaustion. The burdens that I carry weigh my spirit down. Sometimes I feel as if I cannot take even one more step.

O Lord, when I grow tired, refresh me. When the sacrifices I make to follow you seem too much, set my heart aflame with the love that bears all things. Teach me to embrace the cross of your choosing, and not to seek what I would choose. As I carry your presence in my heart, help me to bear you to the world — even as you have borne me up to heaven.

Amen.

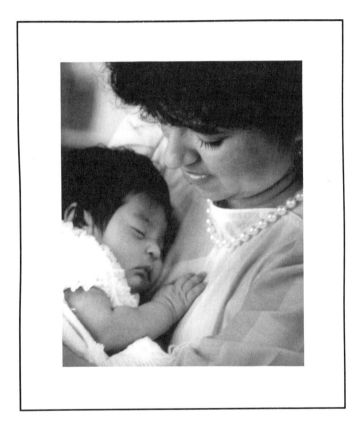

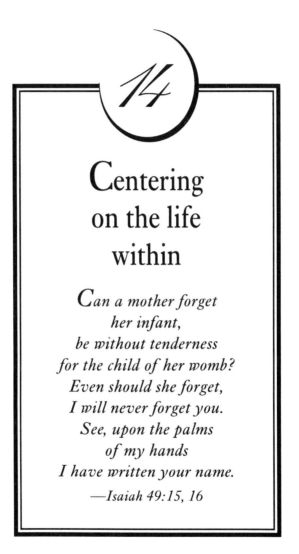

14

Centering on the life within

Can a mother forget
her infant,
be without tenderness
for the child of her womb?
Even should she forget,
I will never forget you.
See, upon the palms
of my hands
I have written your name.

—Isaiah 49:15, 16

It's funny how when you have a new baby, it seems that you've had her all your life. From the minute I first knew about each of our children, I could think of nothing else. Every waking moment — and many sleeping ones as well — were at least punctuated, if not dominated, by thoughts of the little stranger inside.

Regardless of what I was doing, "the baby" always took center stage. Mentally, I'd maintain huge lists of all the things I needed to do. I'd interrupt myself to move the furniture around in order to gain more space, and then usually put it back the way it was. Regular responsibilities took a back seat to sorting through clothes and toys with a vengeance. Priorities and schedules shifted to accommodate things that I had to get done B.B. — "Before Baby."

A strong sense of urgency always made me feel like there was something I had forgotten, or was about to forget. Never realizing just how preoccupied I was with the impending new arrival, I made all kinds of unconscious accommodations. At the end of my first two pregnancies, I remember thinking that it would be wise not to start the laundry because it might be interrupted by labor. If I had continued with that line of reasoning, I would have had a month-high pile of dirty clothes to wash after I returned home from the hospital. Thankfully, I came to my senses.

During pregnancy not just our bodies, but our whole selves are busy tending to the new life within us. While our physical resources are focused on an unborn baby, our thoughts and feelings become captivated by his presence. We naturally begin to live our lives with reference to the someone else that is there.

Likewise, our babies are captivated by us. For unlike the photographs that occasionally grace the covers of magazines, an unborn child is not suspended in space. His whole world is his mother. Everything he can experience is filtered through her.

This mutual absorption extends to the entire family. Older children make preparations of their own, and even fathers make plans. Whether with joy or anxiety, new life quickly becomes the focus of our concerns.

Sadly, however, our preparations remain primarily material. We buy our diapers and clothes. We set up our cribs. We make decisions about feeding and about our use of time and money. We do all the things that need to be done. Most of us prepare for a birth like we do for Christmas, frantically baking and decorating, shopping and wrapping packages until the day comes. But when it comes, even though everything is done, we feel that we have missed something.

With later pregnancies, I've begun to wonder whether those indispensable and urgent necessities really prepare our family at all. I have come to the conclusion that, somehow, all that stuff gets done anyway; and that it's no sin to set up a crib while I'm in the hospital. No doubt, the diapers are important. But more important than the diapers, is creating the spiritual and emotional readiness to welcome a new baby home. These are deeper preparations.

The scriptures tell us precious little about the plans Mary made for the birth of her Son. Certainly, there were fewer options, and fewer choices to be made. Mary didn't have to decide between bottle or breast, cloth or disposable, "natural" or with anesthesia. But what has always surprised me, is that she doesn't appear to have made arrangements in Bethlehem for the birth itself!

It could appear that Mary was not a well-organized young mother. Nevertheless, I think that she was more prepared for the birth of her child than most of us have ever been for ours. When Mary says, "Behold, I am the handmaid of the Lord" (Luke 1:38), it is clear that she has prepared her heart.

Mary was ready to receive what God would give because her life was centered on him. Jesus had been the focus of her thoughts, and emotions, and choices all along. Now her material existence would be centered on him as well. Mary was prepared for anything. We hear it in her voice when she says, "May it be done to me according to your word" (Luke 1:38).

While we can only guess at Mary's preparations, the accounts of God's preparations for the birth of Christ are innumerable. Through prophets and kings, by law and sacrifice, in slavery, exile, and persecution, God had carefully planned his coming. The entire history of humankind records God's work to prepare not only a virgin, but a people, and a world to receive his Son.

But it is not the birth of Jesus in Bethlehem for which God prepared. There was no room in Bethlehem, because that is not the room God had been preparing. Jesus did not come to be born in an inn or a stable, but in our hearts. God did not shower his attentions on Jesus, but on us. His love, though centered *in* Christ, centers *on* us.

It's almost comic to think of a pregnant woman forgetting the baby she carries. (No one who sees her does!) We all know that even when we try, it's nearly impossible to ignore the presence of another person in the same room once we know they're there. Yet, it seems so easy to forget the God who dwells in our hearts.

We sense one another's presence every day. Intimacy, whether with an unborn child, with one another, or with God, depends on what we do with the presence we sense. We may not be able to ignore another person, but we can limit the intimacy of our encounters. We can choose to be more "alongside" others, than "with" them.

Knowing that God centers himself on us, Mary centered herself on him. Our faith calls us to do the same. We are so easily absorbed by the presence of a child in the womb. But we must learn to be captivated by the divine presence that stirs in our hearts. There are too many distractions to the life of faith. To center ourselves on the interior life of the Spirit, rather than on the exterior life that surrounds us, is to choose the better part.

———————————

O God, beneath the thin crust that forms the surface of my life, you are ever present. On my right and on my left, above and below, before and behind, you surround me with your love. Within my very heart, you dwell with me always.

But, Lord, I give so much of my attention to what is shallow. I sometimes try to ignore you, and go about my business as if you weren't even there. And, when I seek you, I look everywhere but in my own soul.

Lord, teach me to live my life with reverence to you alone. Help me to enter within my soul, and teach me to find you at the very center of my heart. Steal me away from all distractions and captivate me. Prepare my life to receive you, and help me to choose you over all else.

Amen.

———————————

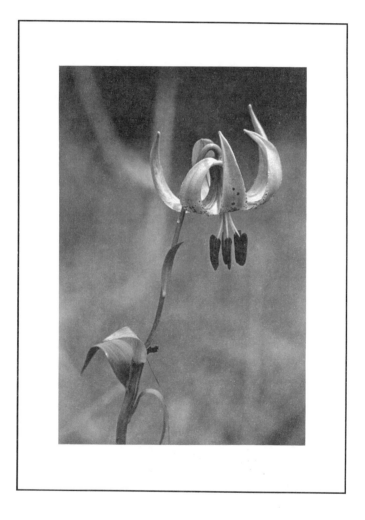

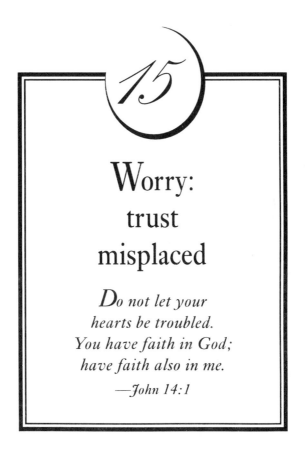

15

Worry: trust misplaced

Do not let your hearts be troubled. You have faith in God; have faith also in me.

—*John 14:1*

I remember waking up late one morning shortly after bringing our first baby home. Looking at the clock, I thought something had to be wrong. I hadn't been disturbed all night, and the baby should have been up three hours before! What in the world happened?

Fearing the worst, I ran to the crib to see if she was still alive and breathing. My heart was thumping. I felt like I had been caught up in a whirlwind. But when I got to the crib, I found the baby blissfully asleep. All she had done was sleep through the night.

A small irregularity had flipped the switch of my imagination. But once hysteria exploded, it seemed to have a life of its own. You'd think that I would have learned from that experience. But I have to admit that I have repeated that scene with each of our four children.

Sometimes, though, there is real cause for concern. When I was five months along with our son, a speeding drunk driver hit our car. The impact was so great that our hats and shoes flew off our heads and feet. The glass from our rear window was shattered on the street. My two girls seemed alright, but we were all very shook up. All I could think about was losing my baby.

When the ambulance came, we were put on boards, and rushed to emergency. For the sake of the girls, I knew I had to act calmly even if I wasn't really calm. But hearing that little heart beating regularly on the monitor flooded me with tears of relief. Except for some sore necks and backs, all of us were fine.

Worry was something quite new to me. I had been a rather carefree child growing up. It had always bothered me to see how much anxiety my mother had. I often vowed to myself, (loud enough for my mother to hear), that I would never become a "worrywart." That was a promise easy to keep — until I became a mother myself.

Worry seems to be part of a mother's job description. In wanting the best for our children, we find plenty of things to be anxious about. But whether the circumstances that prompt our anxiety are justified or not, the underlying reason is the same. We worry about situations we cannot

control. We often end up becoming out of control ourselves.

Most of us live our daily lives acting as if we are sitting
in the driver's seat. Even if we know how short our reach
is, we're still shocked when something happens to us that
is beyond our control. The fact is, that we deeply desire to
run our own lives. Anything that flies in the face of that
desire causes us great consternation.

It's tempting to think that Mary had nothing to worry
about. After all, her son was the Son of God. Surely, God
would take care of everything. But when we look at what
we know about Mary's life, it is clear that she did not
"have it made" by any stretch of the imagination.

On the contrary, Mary had at least as much to worry
about as her contemporaries did — and certainly more
than we do. To begin with, she lived in a time and culture
that did not welcome unwed mothers with open arms, but
with stones in hand. Being pregnant under those circumstances was a definite cause for anxiety. Mary would have
a lot of explaining to do, to Joseph and her own family as
well. Even if Joseph didn't have the heart to stone her, he
may not have had the heart to take her into his house
either.

Without a man to provide for her, Mary would be desti-
tute. Even widows, if they had no sons, were left with no
financial standing whatsoever. A woman's social position
was entirely dependent on the status of the man who cared
for her. Mary would not have been able to support herself.
No one would have done business with her.

Mary had absolutely no control over the circumstances
of her life, but she did not respond with anxiety or fear.
Mary knew better than to worry about what she could not

control. She did not entrust her well-being to a man, or to her own ingenuity. Difficult circumstances swirled around her, but she was not overcome with grief. Rather, she rested secure in the hand of God. She knew that God was in control. He would not let her down.

We all know that worry accomplishes nothing. Nevertheless, we spend a great deal of ourselves in nervous desperation. When we worry, it's not because we don't trust anything, but because we have trusted the wrong thing. Perhaps we have relied on a check in the mail, a medical exam, a family member, or even ourselves. Anxiety erupts when we trust in anything other than God.

Anxiety poisons our lives. It steals our joy and our freedom; it fosters discontent — it can even make us physically ill. Moreover, it undermines our faith by convincing us that God is neither powerful nor faithful.

Worry tells us to take over the wheel, but God invites us to sit back and enjoy the ride. He begs us to look at the lilies of the field, and the birds of the air. They do not toil or spin, they do not sow or reap; and yet, he cares for them (Matthew 6:26, 28). He asks us to consider what it would be like if we did control our own lives. Perhaps, on second thought, it would be more frightening than allowing God to do so.

The cure for anxiety is prayer. The scriptures teach us that while we should "be anxious for nothing" (Philippians 4:6), we should "pray without ceasing" (1 Thessalonians 5:17). God promises us his peace, not when we struggle to hold on to life with a death grip, but when we allow him to hold us in his loving arms.

God encourages us not to worry for our children, but to pray for them. He assures us that when we are not in control, he is. He tells us that all we need do is ask, seek, and knock — to come to him in confidence with every burden. There is nothing that is beyond the power of his love. Instead of misplacing trust in our own lives, how much wiser it is to place our trust in the source of all life.

O Lord, how self-sufficient and independent I think I am! How foolishly I pretend that I can plan every step I take, and author every chapter of my life! How readily I ride life like a horse, believing that I hold the reins!

But when the facade falls around me, and I can no longer trust in myself, I find it difficult to trust in you. The storms that rage around me also rage within me. I am overcome with anxiety and fear. I spend my days in anguish and my nights in sleepless distress. The reality of my powerlessness frightens me.

Teach me, O God, to know my weakness, so that I may learn to know your strength. Show me that there is nothing beyond your reach. Pull every false support out from under me, until I place my life completely in your hands. Keep me at rest in the power of your faithfulness. Teach me to be anxious for nothing and to pray without ceasing.

Amen.

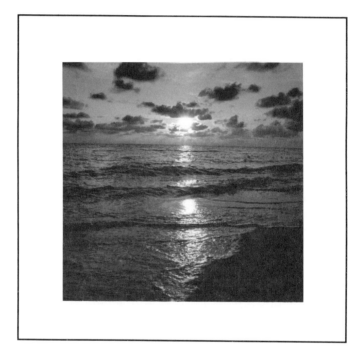

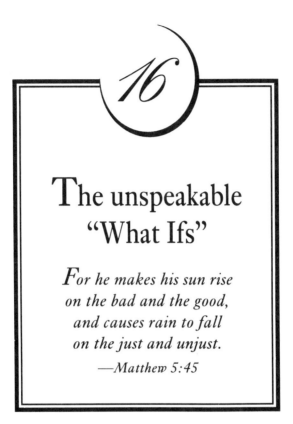

16

The unspeakable "What Ifs"

*For he makes his sun rise
on the bad and the good,
and causes rain to fall
on the just and unjust.*

—*Matthew 5:45*

Although I don't remember ever discussing my concerns for the health of my children out loud, I do recall a series of nightmares I had during my first pregnancy. In these dreams my baby would be born prematurely, and then be diagnosed with some terrible condition. One night it would be Down's syndrome, another spina bifida, or cerebral palsy. Over the course of a few weeks, I went through almost every illness I could name.

The dreams were so vivid, I began to wonder if they were premonitions. To make it worse, almost every conversation I had about my baby seemed to end with the same refrain. Boy or girl, cute or ugly, gifted or just one of the crowd, nothing mattered "as long as it's healthy!"

But what if my baby wasn't healthy? What if there was something wrong — even something seriously wrong? I began to ask myself just what I'd do, and how I'd feel, if my baby wasn't "normal." I wasn't sure that I liked my answers much at all.

Most of us wonder if our children will be healthy, and if not, we wonder what we will do. We all hope for the best, but at the same time we know that for some mothers, these hopes will be in vain. For the most part, our fears remain unvoiced.

It isn't pleasant to think about the lives of families with children who are not well. While we admire their courage, most of us keep our distance. We do everything we can to hold onto the belief that it can't happen to us. We tell ourselves that the deck is stacked in our favor. After all, those things only happen to people who can handle them.

Suffering makes us uncomfortable. It seems beyond our grasp to understand or explain it. But in particular, a child who suffers presents us with a most acute dilemma. We shake our fists at heaven when we see a child in pain.

Realizing how much we take for granted, most of us are rather ungrateful. At some level, we all think we deserve nothing less than a "perfect" child. The fact is that no child is "perfect." We can deceive ourselves about some longer than we can about others, but human limitation eventually catches up with all of us. As important as good health is, it is not a ticket to a life without difficulties.

Most of us would agree that we deserve suffering no more than we deserve blessing. But underneath it all, we hear a voice telling us that if there is something wrong, we are somehow to blame. Many of us often connect suffering with sin. We tend to think of it as some kind of divine payback — a deserved sentence for a committed offense. Like those followers of Jesus who encountered the man born blind, we ask "Who sinned, this man or his parents?" (John 9:2).

But what are we saying about God when we insist on seeing things from this point of view? Surely a loving Father would not send suffering upon his children! Certainly, if God was all-powerful, he would not stand by and allow a child, life's greatest joy, to become life's greatest burden. We get even more perplexed when we notice that these terrible things seem to happen to all the wrong people.

Most of us respond to suffering in our lives with a shout of "Why me?" Perhaps the deepest answer to that question is the one that is the simplest — "Why not?" No one is exempt from pain. No matter how good someone may seem to have it, rest assured, everyone has a load to bear. The cross always looks lighter when someone else is carrying it.

Suffering tempts us to give it more power over us than it actually has. We do so by letting it distort and dominate our perspective. A child with an illness has a set of difficulties others may not have. But whatever the diagnosis is, we don't give birth to problems, but to children. The problems may be terrible, but the child is always good.

The particular challenges we may face with a child who is ill do not have to interfere with our love for them. At root, and no matter how sick a child is, the human capacity to love and be loved remains constant. The quality of a person's life is more determined by the quality of the person, than by the quality of the life.

While suffering disturbs us at the deepest levels, it is important that we make peace with it. Our faith teaches us that in our trials there is not only the hidden presence of God, but a hidden purpose in the pain. We want to believe that suffering somehow makes sense. Christian discipleship assures us that it does.

As difficult as it is to accept our hardships and those of our children, we must remember that God's only Son wasn't spared either. If anyone in history didn't deserve it, it was Jesus. Nonetheless, his whole mission, the redemption of the world, was accomplished through suffering.

Both God and Mary shared that suffering. Mary felt the sword pierce her heart as any mother would. But she was able to stand at the cross because God's grace flowed from it. And, because ultimately, the fruit of that tree was not death, but life.

The cross of Christ makes clear to us that suffering never comes alone. When it comes, it is always accompanied by the grace to bear it, and a gift to rejoice in it. Strange as it may seem, we call that awful day of crucifixion "Good Friday." We do so because we have found wrapped in the greatest suffering imaginable, a gift beyond imagination.

An unhealthy child is not a gift anyone would choose. Nonetheless, every child remains a gift. Most of us have heard the parents of children with poor medical prognoses express how those children have enriched their lives. They show us that it is possible to look beyond the illness, because there is something — or someone — beyond it.

show us that it is possible to look beyond the illness, because there is something — or someone — beyond it.

The cross is not a place where any of us want to be. But at the cross, we may begin to understand the answer Jesus gave regarding suffering. To those who asked about the man born blind he said, "Neither he nor his parents sinned; it is so that works of God might be made visible through him" (John 9:3).

━━━━━━━━━━━

Lord, there are so many things I take for granted, and so many blessings I have left uncounted. I have gone about so much of my life expecting fairy-tale endings, and happily-ever-afters. I am convinced that I deserve nothing less.

Yet underneath it all, I know how frail life can be, and how even small matters cast long shadows. Afraid of what suffering challenges me to bear, I run away from what it offers me. I am all too ready to take the blame, yet far too hesitant to accept the cross.

Lord, help me to see that in suffering lies redemption. Reveal to me, O God, the glory that is hidden there, and teach me to look beyond the suffering into your compassionate face.

Amen.

━━━━━━━━━━━

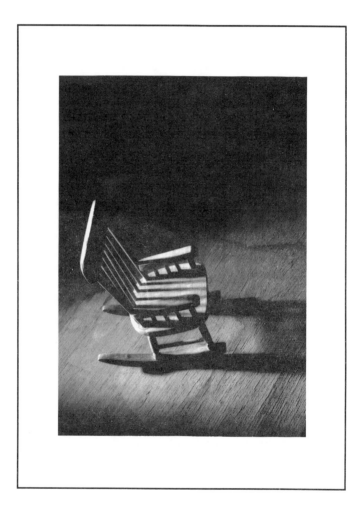

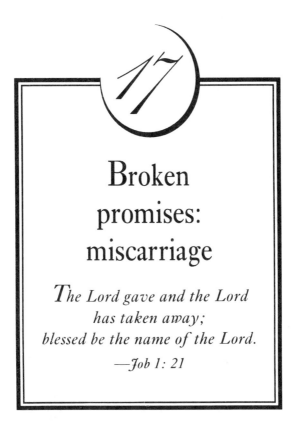

Broken promises: miscarriage

*The Lord gave and the Lord
has taken away;
blessed be the name of the Lord.*

—*Job 1: 21*

If having a child is one of our greatest joys, losing a child is as great a sorrow. Although we don't like to think about it, not every pregnancy ends with birth. Most women experience a miscarriage sometime during their reproductive years.

I remember the date of my miscarriage more readily than I do the birth dates of my children. It happened two months into my third pregnancy. I went to the airport to pick up a friend who was visiting for the weekend. When I stopped at the bathroom, I discovered that I was bleeding.

Shaking and crying, I ran to a telephone to call my husband at work. I immediately left for home. He called the doctor, and picked up our friend at the airport. I knew every pregnancy was different, but nothing like this had ever happened to me before.

I stayed in bed, hoping the bleeding would stop, or at least slow down. My doctor met us at the hospital the next morning. He told me that I had to wait it out, but that I hadn't lost the baby yet. He also told me that if I did miscarry, I would know it. The chances were about fifty-fifty.

I did everything I could think of to save my baby. I stayed in bed. I spent a lot of time on the phone consulting a friend who had been through a miscarriage the previous month. I tried to stay positive and muster all the hope I could. I did a lot of praying.

My physical condition did improve a little, but my emotional state continued to deteriorate. I felt as if I was in a constant state of emergency. The siren had sounded, and the bell had rung, but there was nothing I could do to stop whatever was happening.

While the alarm continued to ring in my ears, everyone around me seemed calm. For them, time would tell. But for me, the turmoil and the waiting were more than I could stand.

A few days later, my doctor scheduled an ultrasound. I had never had one with my other two pregnancies, so I wasn't sure what to expect. He told me that what we were hoping to find was a "smudge" with a beat.

During the procedure, the technician seemed puzzled. When my doctor called later that day, I found out why.

The sonogram showed absolutely no sign of pregnancy. My womb was empty and clean. There wasn't any need for a D & C. I had, in fact, miscarried. The baby was gone, and so was the hope I had held on to.

The pain of that loss did not draw our family together. Rather, each of us sought his own means of coping with it. I knew that my husband and children were deeply disappointed. Nevertheless, they all seemed able to accept it. Knowing that I had miscarried was not the resolution they wanted; but for them, it was a resolution nonetheless. The pregnancy was over, and the miscarriage was over too.

For me, however, the grief had just begun. There were no mixed emotions or feelings for me to sort out. There was just sadness, deep sadness like an aching emptiness nothing could relieve. I knew that my baby hadn't just disappeared. He had died. And worse, it had happened inside me.

I kept thinking that everything would be better "tomorrow," but "tomorrow" never came. Everyone expected that I would get over it. But every time I saw a pregnant woman, the wound opened up all over again. I'm sure I never saw so many pregnant women in my life. It seemed like they had all come out of the woodwork just to spite me. I was angry at God for allowing the miscarriage to happen. Now it seemed as though he was adding insult to injury.

Whatever I did, I could not get out from under the lonely cloud that hung over me. Despite the well-intentioned people who tried to comfort me, I felt completely alone. They encouraged me to be grateful for the children I already had. Many told me that it was all a "blessing in disguise"; that probably something had been very wrong with my baby anyway. They reminded me that I was young, and was sure to get pregnant again. None of what people said to me helped. For the most part, I think it made things worse.

It seemed that no one was willing to treat my miscarriage like what it actually was — the loss of a child. Of course I was grateful for the daughters I already had. If anything, the miscarriage had made me more grateful, not less. And I knew that my baby may have had serious problems that caused the miscarriage. The pain, however, wasn't any less real. He was mine, and I already loved him. I also knew that I might well have other children in the future. But that is what they'd be, other children. This child, this individual, was lost to me forever.

I don't know what it's like to lose a child who has already lived as a part of the family. Most of us have not even seen the unborn children we have lost, let alone held them, cared for them, or enjoyed them as individuals. Many seem to think that this relative detachment lessens the loss. But in my own experience of miscarriage, it was precisely these unfulfilled expectations—these broken promises—that hurt most.

Days passed, but I couldn't stop crying. I didn't weep for the loss of a relationship I had, but for one I would never have. The grief I experienced was rooted in what might have been — what should have been—not in what was. I regretted that my baby and I would never have the chance to become to each other what we were meant to be.

Having nowhere else to turn, I began to pray again. Because it no longer made sense to pray for my baby, I began to ask my baby to pray with me. I was convinced that I had been carrying a boy, so I named him Paul. I poured out my grief to him and to God over what had happened. I told him that I loved him, that I had wanted him very much, and that I missed him terribly. I trusted that he was with God. Finally, the darkness began to vanish.

Although it was true that my baby was gone, I realized that I had let the miscarriage rob me of more than that. My pain had eclipsed the relationship I had with my lost child. I had allowed myself to experience the reality of the loss, but had distanced myself from the reality of the child.

The intensity of the loss had made everything seem like such a waste. But when I pursued my child spiritually — when I dared to seek him out — the value of his life became apparent. Naming my baby, and praying with him, preserved the relationship that death could not steal. Suddenly, Paul's life became more to me than just the few weeks he had lived inside me. He was more than a miscarriage, a mistake, or a footnote. He was a child of mine alive in the presence of the God who had created him.

However short his life was, I began to understand that Paul was God's gift to me just as my other children were. The quality of the gift was not diminished by the fact that we had so little time together. We belonged to one another for all eternity. Our joy in heaven would be the greater because of our loss on earth.

Losing Paul taught me that God is faithful; that God does not break his promises. Even in the midst of the pain and disappointment of what looked like an unfulfilled promise of new life, God was there. God is with us and for us. He is never lost to us. Sickness and death may snatch us away from one another, but nothing can snatch us out of his hand. He is forever showing us that even in loss, there is gain.

O Lord, you are gracious to me beyond measure. You shower me with good gifts. You withhold nothing from me. You fill my cup to overflowing. Perhaps that is why it is so hard for me to accept loss.

But Lord, you are a God with two hands: one that gives, and one that takes away. You give freely so that I might learn to freely receive; and you take so that I might learn to give.

Father, do not let the pain of loss isolate me from others or from you. Rather use it to draw me ever closer to your heart; to hold you even more dear than what you have given—or what you have seen fit to take away. Show me that what I lose is only for a time, but that what I gain in you is eternal. For all things are passing, Lord, except you. And though I lose everything, possessing you alone, I possess all there is.

Amen.

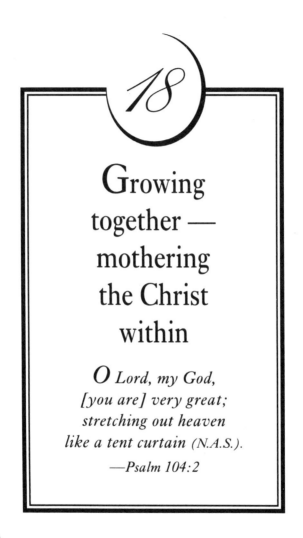

18

Growing together — mothering the Christ within

O Lord, my God, [you are] very great; stretching out heaven like a tent curtain (N.A.S.).

—Psalm 104:2

At my very first visit to the obstetrician, I was told that my bone structure made me a good candidate for cesarean delivery. According to my doctor, any baby much over seven pounds could prove beyond my ability to deliver naturally. Believing that God and nature did a pretty good job taking care of these things, I wasn't particularly upset. The fact that I had weighed under six pounds at birth myself, gave me reason to expect a small baby. I figured that I had little cause for concern.

What I didn't realize, though, was just how big any baby really is. When they are newborns, even the big ones look small — but before they are born, even the small ones are quite sizable. To my surprise, it wasn't too long before I filled what had seemed like unnecessary room in my maternity clothes. Both my baby and I grew at breakneck speed. The baby stretched to fill all the available space, and I stretched to make more space available.

It wasn't just my belly that got bigger. Everything grew: my arms and ankles, face, and even my feet. In fact, having always had a rather girlish figure, it was quite shocking for me to go up three bra sizes in just six weeks!

All that stretching did not come without pain or discomfort. Muscles I didn't know I had ached under the stress. Discovering heartburn, water retention, and stretch marks, I couldn't help but wonder just how much anyone could stretch before bursting at the seams! Nonetheless, when all was said and done, I delivered our first daughter at nine pounds and eleven ounces — without a cesarean section.

My body, however, wasn't the only thing that needed to be stretched. Obviously, my baby depended on my physical ability to stretch to accommodate her as she grew. But far beyond the nine months before birth, she would depend on me to stretch my heart for her as well. I would have to learn to nurture her not just with my body, but with my whole life.

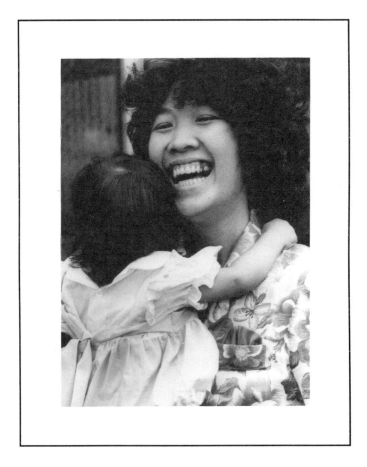

Maternity stretches a woman inside and out. While our bodies grow openly and publicly, our hearts do so in secret. The inner stretches of the soul are neither less astonishing, nor less painful, than the outward and more visible ones. But unlike the swelling of the womb with child, most of the growth we experience is not temporary or passing. We are forever altered by it. We are never again the same as before. After five pregnancies, I know that for me single-digit dress sizes are probably gone forever. It is my hope, however, that single-digit soul sizes are gone as well.

Love requires us to stretch for one another. The call to expand our hearts is not for mothers only. It resounds in every family as a whole. With each new addition, parents must learn to split their energies, and older children must learn to share and to wait. Most families with more than one child know how difficult these lessons can be. But it seems that children have an special elasticity of spirit. I have seen few things more beautiful to watch than an older sister kissing her younger brother's bruised knee, or a baby at home running to the door to greet the older children as they return from school. Families are, indeed, where we learn to love.

As the days and weeks of Mary's pregnancy passed, she blossomed just like the rest of us. Her young body, filled with new life, had to stretch to accommodate her child. But Mary's heart, and her life, had to expand even more. Her pregnancy, after all, was like no other pregnancy before. Nor was her child just any child. For this obscure and provincial teen-ager, life would change dramatically. This child would bring her both attention and adversity. Because of him Mary would travel to Bethlehem, escape to Egypt, settle in Galilee, and ultimately, stand beneath a cross. Through it all, Mary stretched and grew. For as the scriptures tell us, she "treasured all these things in her heart" (Luke 2: 51 N.A.S.).

At first glance, the significance of that one day of the annunciation seems to take on enormous proportion. It is tempting to identify the angel's visit as the obvious turning point which would define and direct Mary's life. But to do so would be to ignore the secret inner life of Mary's soul that brought her there. What changed Mary's life was not simply a single moment or event, but the unparalleled intimacy she shared with God so clearly reflected in that moment.

Mary's relationship with God did not begin with the angel's message, nor by becoming the mother of the Son. It was because she had mothered and nurtured his Spirit in her heart, that Mary fulfilled God's purpose for her life. His presence grew in her soul, long before and long after he grew as a child in her womb.

It is not Mary's, but our intimacy with God that has its beginnings in the annunciation. Through her willingness to open her life to the Son of God, Mary brought Jesus to us. Further, her life of grace shows us what it means to be stretched and formed by the indwelling presence of the Divine Stranger. Because Mary centered her life on nurturing his life within her, God was not a stranger.

People, and not things, both cause and enable our personal growth. They are often the source of our greatest challenge, as well as our deepest joy. But we do not accord everyone in our lives equal influence. We don't stretch for a stranger like we do for a friend; nor for a friend like we do for a family member. Intimacy determines the degree to which someone will be able to shape and foster our growth. Our bodies stretch for our unborn children because they are inside us. Our hearts and lives stretch for them because our children reach to the core of our inner beings.

Although bearing the child Jesus was a privilege reserved for Mary alone, like Mary, we all bear his presence in the womb of our hearts. We know that a child in the womb cannot sustain growth and development without our nurturing and mothering him. Most of us do everything we can to assure that our unborn children are being nurtured properly.

But somehow, many of us lose sight of the need to nurture the Christ in our hearts. We focus so exclusively on our identity as children of God, that we do not allow ourselves to mother the divine life God plants within us. We must learn to feed the life of Christ with our own lives, just as we feed our unborn children with our own bodies.

The life of faith is a life of growth. As our children grow to fill more and more of our bodies and lives, so Christ longs to fill our hearts. If we think that we are too small to bear the God who cannot be contained by heaven and earth, we are right. But the intimacy God seeks stretches and expands us. As we mother his growth in us, he will swell our hearts until they are big enough to embrace him fully.

Lord, how great you are indeed! How deep, and how high, and how vast! There is no created thing big enough to hold you, for in just one hand you hold all things. Yet your greatness, Lord, seeks out the small. Your love for the poor and weak draws you to me.

But Lord, I am too small to be your home. Whatever space I have is cramped full of myself. My soul is crowded by worldly concerns. My mind is frenzied with distraction of every kind; and my life is cluttered with vain and useless pursuits.

Stretch me, O God, and swell my heart. Make me the tent of your dwelling. Empty my soul of all that keeps me from you. Teach me to water the seed you have planted, and to feed your life within me with my own. Shape me, O Lord, and mold me from within. Grow in my heart and fill me, until I can contain you no more.

Amen.

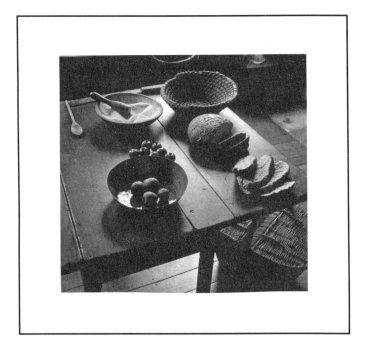

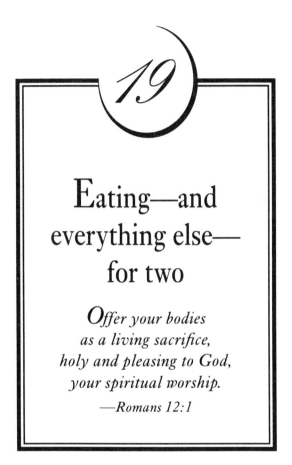

19

Eating—and everything else— for two

Offer your bodies
as a living sacrifice,
holy and pleasing to God,
your spiritual worship.

—*Romans 12:1*

One summer afternoon shortly before we knew we were expecting our son, I came home from my weekly trip to the grocery store. As I set about unpacking the bags, our two girls began to giggle and laugh. I couldn't imagine what was so funny about groceries, until I saw that the kitchen table was filled with lime gelatin, lime sherbet, limeade mix, and fresh limes. I hadn't intended to buy all those lime things. Nonetheless, there they were! There was something strangely familiar about that kind of irrational behavior, but I couldn't put my finger on what it was. A few weeks later, however, the pieces fell into place and we all knew why I had been feeling a little green!

Most of us have stories to tell about what we eat during pregnancy. The cravings we commonly experience always seem to come out of the blue. But when they hit, they are an inescapable force to be reckoned with. I remember waking up one morning with Stove Top stuffing on my mind. Hoping it would pass, I tried to go about my daily routine. Nevertheless, no matter what I did, I just couldn't stop thinking about stuffing. I tried to stave it off by eating lots of carrot sticks. I crusaded against excessive self-indulgence, but to no avail. By supper time, it had become so intense that I finally broke down and consumed a virtual mountain of Stove Top.

Our dietary exploits during pregnancy often involve the quantity of what we eat as well as the quality. One would think that a woman with child would have less room in her stomach for food. But I, for one, have never been able to pack it in like I can when I'm pregnant. Many of us absolutely dread stepping on that merciless scale month after month. I always tried to soften the blow by deducting a generous allowance for my clothing. But despite my sometimes valiant efforts to limit what and how much I ate, at my doctor's office, I hold the record for weight gain in a single month at fourteen pounds. (Not even my biggest baby weighed that much!)

Humorous as they may be, maternal cravings serve a purpose. They are a concrete expression of our children's needs. I didn't need the limes or carrots — and certainly not six servings of stuffing — but somehow, the baby inside me did. Mysteriously and without a voice, she communicated her needs to me, and filled them through me. And regardless of my children's giggles, my husband's raised eyebrows, or my doctor's scale, I could easily justify exotic foods and enormous portions. After all, I was "eating for two."

The fact is, that when we're pregnant we do much more than just eat for two. We breathe, rest, plan, prepare, and hopefully, pray for two as well. Indeed, we actually live for two. Our children cannot care for themselves, so we do most of what they need for them. But if we are to meet our children's physical, emotional, and spiritual needs, we must give not only our bodies, but more importantly, our lives, for our children. We must sacrifice our wants for the sake of their needs.

Although all sacrifice is a kind of death, we are not like the animals once offered on temple altars. We do not die for our children, we live for them. We cannot fulfill our love for them with a single act, but perpetually, with thousands upon thousands of small self-denials that fill a lifetime. We make our whole lives a gift to our children. And in so doing, we become living sacrifices for them.

Although many of us like to think of ourselves as independent and self-reliant, in truth we are not much different from our unborn children. In struggling to provide for our children, we invariably discover that we are unable to provide for all of our own needs. Even those who are the most successful at supplying material necessities, are often at a loss when it comes to filling the emotional or spiritual hungers we share.

Common to each of us is a hunger for something more, something else, something deep. We may not know what — or rather who — we need. We may not even know that we need anything or anyone at all. But in some way, all of us exhibit that inner restlessness of spirit. Those who deny the hunger of the heart starve their souls. Those who perceive it, often don't know how to address it. But whether we choose to ignore or address our spiritual needs, they do not go unexpressed in our lives.

Frequently, the inner cravings of the soul are articulated in the spiritual equivalents of pickles and ice cream. Many, who do not understand the nature of our inner needs, attempt to address them by sampling the full range of exotic "spiritual" experiences. Others attempt to substitute what they cannot supply, with vast quantities of the material things that they are able to acquire for themselves. Ultimately, though, we all find that we cannot be satisfied by our own poor efforts. Just as when we crave one food and try to satisfy it with another, we are left empty.

It is in Christ alone, and through him, that all our needs can be expressed, and filled. Just as the child in the womb must rely on his mother to give voice to his needs, Jesus intercedes for us in the spirit, "with inexpressible groanings"(Romans 8:26). As every child is dependent on his parents to provide for his well-being, so too are we completely dependent on the Lord. He knows that we are too weak to care for our souls. He understands that we cannot supply ourselves with what we need, simply because our deepest need is for him.

Our lives are not our own. Family life teaches us that we belong to one another, and that we depend upon one another. Similarly, our hearts are not just ours. Our spirits are restless precisely because we are made not only by God, but for God. We cry out from the bottomless pit of our human hearts because only God can satisfy our hearts.

We can do nothing to acquire God for ourselves. Yet, he is always ready to give himself to us. We give our children what that they need from our bodies and our lives. Similarly, God gives everything to those who ask — and a great deal to those who don't bother. Jesus tells us that our heavenly Father knows what we need, even before we ask. He teaches us not to worry for food or clothing or shelter. Again and again God promises to "supply whatever you need in accord with his glorious riches"(Philippians 4:19).

Nevertheless, the life of faith is not a one-way street where we ask and receive, and where God listens and gives. For although God is without need, he is not without desires. God hungers for intimacy. The very existence of creation expresses this divine longing. In the beginning, God made all things for himself. God created man and woman in his image to be his friends. He desired us even when we rejected his love. And from the moment of our fall from grace, God prepared our salvation to restore the intimacy we had thrown away.

Human need and divine desire meet in the person of Jesus Christ. In him, God became a living and eternal sacrifice for us. He became one of us, so that he might become one with us. God's desire for intimacy, not ours, leads and directs us deeper in faith. Like the child in the womb who motivates us to do what we must to fill his needs, it is Christ alive in our hearts that moves us closer to him. There is nothing that can take his place in our lives; neither is there anything that can take our place with him. No tree or ocean or mountain can satisfy God's craving for intimacy with every man and woman. Only our hearts can fill the hunger of Christ.

—————

Lord, it is good that you know all our needs even before we ask. For if I came to you with all of them, my prayer would never end! I am completely dependent on your loving kindness. My home, my food, my family, my work—all of these are from you.

Yet, Lord, my restless heart betrays a deeper need. My soul thirsts within me. My flesh craves the something more that I cannot grasp for myself.

Give me yourself, Lord, for I cannot take you. Give me yourself, lest my soul starve. More than food and shelter, Lord, strengthen my faith. Teach me to embrace you not only in need, but in love. Let me desire you as you desire me, that I might fill your hunger, and satisfy your longing.

Amen.

—————

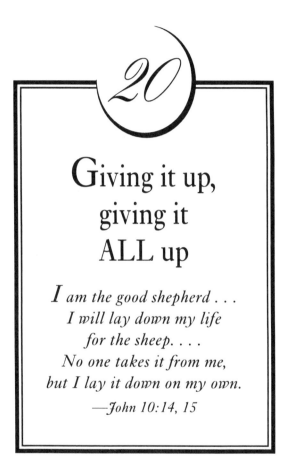

20

Giving it up,
giving it
ALL up

I am the good shepherd . . .
I will lay down my life
for the sheep. . . .
No one takes it from me,
but I lay it down on my own.
—*John 10:14, 15*

When I graduated from college, I had every intention of pursuing a graduate or professional degree of some kind. I was newly married, living far away from anyone I knew, and wasn't exactly sure what direction I ought to take. Under the circumstances, I thought it would be best to take a year off from studies to adjust to my new station in life. I needed time to fully consider my options and goals. I began by collecting information and applications to various graduate programs in the area. I thought carefully, discerning and planning what I would do next. But six months later, when everything began to come into focus, I found out that I was pregnant.

Having a baby was not the next step I had planned to take. Nonetheless, it was wonderfully exciting. The idea didn't upset my apple cart too much. After all, I had known plenty of graduate students who had completed their studies and had a baby too. It wouldn't be easy, but it wasn't impossible either. Nevertheless, I decided to put graduate school on hold until the baby was a year old.

Time flew by. And as our baby approached her first birthday, I pursued the further education I had tabled. But just as I was about to begin the first semester of classes, I conceived again. Needless to say, I was not a happy camper. This time, I was devastated. I knew what it took to care for a child. I also knew that there was little chance of my being able to handle two children and a graduate education of any kind simultaneously. Although I wanted to have more than one child, I also wanted to go on with my own life. I felt as if all my plans were crashing down around me at once. I had to blame it all on something. The baby was the most logical choice.

As difficult as it was for me to adjust to having two children, it was even more difficult to stand by and watch my dreams die. I didn't have to worry any more about what kind of education or career to pursue. The answer was "none." I didn't have to wonder whether I'd be happier as a lawyer or a professor, because I wouldn't be a lawyer or a professor. All I would be was what I already was — a

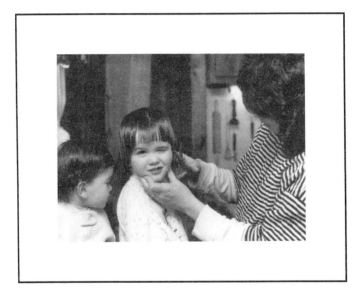

mother. Whatever abilities I had would be buried in a pile of diapers. I felt like Gulliver, tied down and trapped by Lilliputians.

I really loved my two children. Yet underneath that love I nursed and harbored a great deal of resentment. Life hadn't turned out the way I had planned it, and I wasn't even twenty-five. I hadn't accomplished much of anything, and probably never would. I was envious of my husband's ability to develop his skills in the workplace. To make it worse, he was enrolled in a master's program.

The demands of motherhood do make it difficult for a woman to accomplish much in terms of her own personal development. I always get a laugh out of people who tell you to make sure that you have time for yourself. For me, those occasional moments weren't worth the backlog of falling behind in whatever had to be done. Usually by the time the children were in their beds, I was ready to crawl into mine.

It is difficult to resist the conclusion that somehow our children steal something from us. We all expect that raising a family will cost us something in time, energy, and resources. But few of us are prepared to make the sacrifices in personal goals and fulfillment that those glowing little faces ask us to make. Resentment builds. It can become so deep that some of us attempt to live out our aspirations in the lives of our children. Others use their children to absolve themselves from any real attempt to lead an otherwise fruitful and productive life.

Almost all of us await the day when our children are older and we can get back to living our own lives. That day never comes. The reason it never comes is that our children are not interruptions to our lives. They are the substance of our lives. We have all heard the saying "small children — small problems; big children — big problems." From my point of view, I would replace the word "problems" with "sacrifices." Although for the most part we are all willing to make sacrifices for our kids, we seem to hope and think that someday the need to sacrifice will end.

If we take a look at our own lives, we may begin to realize that we ourselves necessitate sacrifice in the lives of those who love us. Indeed, as long as there is love, there will be sacrifice. If we plan to love our children for the rest of our lives, then we must plan to sacrifice for the rest of our lives as well. And, if we wish to love each another without limits, then we must be prepared to place no limits on what we are willing to give up for one another.

The life of Mary is a portrait of loving well. In terms of self-sacrifice, Mary's Son was much more costly to her than most of our children are to us. Few of us would want to trade places with her. By the end of her life, Mary had not only seen it all, she had given it all. It began with giving her humanity to enflesh the Word of God. It ended with her surrendering her soul into God's loving hands.

Like all of us, she was continually challenged to embrace greater and greater sacrifices. Mary's first yes was certainly not her last. To be the mother of the Savior, Mary risked her reputation, her security, her privacy. She had to leave her home, her country, and the rest of her family behind. Whatever ideas she had about how she'd live her life would have to take a back seat to God's plan of salvation. Indeed, Mary's whole identity would be overshadowed and defined by her divine son. She gave up everything for him, living her whole life for the sake of Christ. And if that wasn't enough, in the end, she watched him being given up to crowd and cross as well.

Mary's life was full of hardships, but it was also full of joy. In comparison with Mary, God asks so little from us. Why, then, do our lives of faith seem lacking in joy? I think it is because when we sacrifice something, we do so grudgingly. In trying to obey his will, we may have allowed God to take what he wanted. But we have not yet learned how to give freely. There is no joy in letting someone take from us. But there is abundant joy in giving, especially in sacrificial giving. The scriptures teach us that it was "for the sake of the joy set before him, he [Jesus] endured the cross" (Hebrews 12:2).

The secret Mary knew was that God would exact nothing from her. He would not take, but only give. She understood that she had the power to give her life to him, or to hold it back. Choosing to lay down her life in love, she found great joy.

We possess the very same power to give our lives to God. We all know that no matter how much we give up for our children, we always receive more. We know, too, that we cannot love our children well by giving them only our resources of time and money. We must give ourselves.

In our lives of discipleship the same principle holds true. God will not be outdone in generosity. God gives us not just all of creation, but himself — the Creator — as well. He sacrifices not only all he has, but all he is in love for us. God keeps nothing of what we give to him, for whatever we sacrifice, whatever we give, serves only to multiply his grace toward us. Most of what we long to hang onto merely serves to keep us from him. What we struggle to grasp with our hands, so often steals the joy from our hearts.

———

O God, I treasure all your blessings. You have filled my life with good things to overflowing. You've given me all I have needed and much of what I have desired.

But Lord, I often act as if your blessings are only meant for me — as if I am the sole beneficiary of your gifts. Though you have given to me without limits, I am always limiting how I give to others — even to those I love.

Lord, teach me to give without reservation, without counting the cost, without tabulating the return. Take away my resentment and give me joy. Teach me the art of sacrificial love. In every thing I give up, whether great or small, reveal to me the power of your redemption. Show me that you only take one gift to give another. Help me to choose to lay my life down, to give not only what I have, but what I am to your glory.

Amen.

———

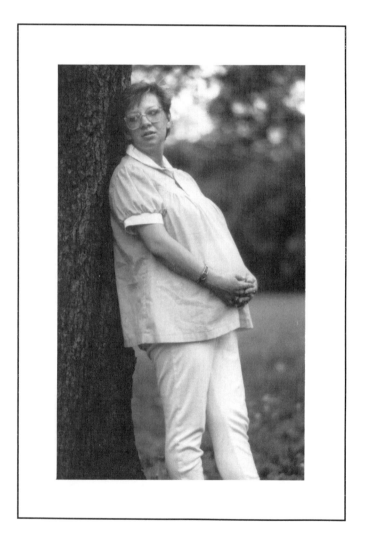

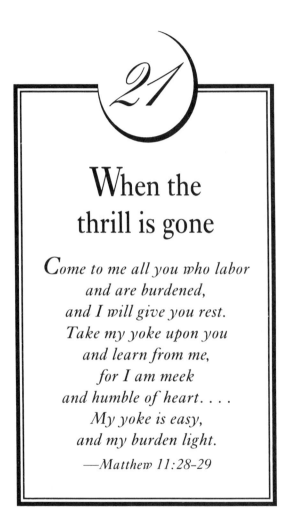

21

When the thrill is gone

Come to me all you who labor
and are burdened,
and I will give you rest.
Take my yoke upon you
and learn from me,
for I am meek
and humble of heart. . . .
My yoke is easy,
and my burden light.
—*Matthew 11:28-29*

Every pregnancy begins with a great deal of excitement. Regardless of whether a woman is expecting her first child or her eighth, new life gives us a thrill. It is like taking a walk in a spring garden at the end of a long winter. There may be nothing new to us about daffodils or tulips, but we find the garden fresh and lovely nonetheless.

Pregnancy was never a secret I could keep. Although there were times that I thought it would be best to delay any announcements, it was never long before I'd be on the phone telling everyone the good news. Like a little girl I played maternity dress-up. I delighted in filling the dresser drawers with little undershirts and tiny socks.

I've noticed that my husband always smiles more when I'm pregnant. (Almost as if he knew something I didn't.) But he isn't the only one who gets into the act. Our two older girls have relished accompanying me to the doctor. They love to hear the pure magic of a new baby's heartbeat. The whole thing opens up a new realm of fantasy for them. During my last two pregnancies, I've caught them stuffing dolls under their dresses, and discussing the relative benefits of nursing or bottle-feeding. For them, especially, maternity has been as delicious as a hot fudge sundae.

It has surprised me that even when I would have rather not been expecting another child, excitement has still been part of each of my pregnancies. In the early weeks, I have always felt like I was walking on air. It is a sensation similar to what many would describe as falling in love. I suppose, in fact, that is exactly what it was — falling in love with a new child. The morning sickness, the weight gain, the exhaustion — none of that seemed important. A new baby was coming! A whole new person was on the way!

But as the weeks and months passed, that romantic air grew stale. Just getting around became a major production.

I could hardly fit behind the driver's wheel, let alone fasten a seat belt. My feet and ankles swelled so much that I found it difficult to walk. The days were full of backaches and heartburn, while restless nights were punctuated by frequent trips to the bathroom. Even though I had plenty of maternity clothes, I never had anything to wear. (I couldn't imagine why I ever thought those big white collars were cute)! And, to top it all off, in three out of five pregnancies, I have broken out in an itchy rash that would drive anyone crazy. Suffice it to say that I got sick and tired of being sick and tired. My family has become rather sick and tired as well.

Maternity is a "gift" many of us would like to return. Most of us would agree that pregnancy and children are a lot of fun. But when we are exhausted, or at the end of our rope, suddenly, the fun is over. The excitement dies down just as the hard work of pregnancy gets harder. Our wonder at the miracle of it all wears very thin. Eventually, the things that were once a source of joy, become a burden.

Interestingly, there is a certain one-upsmanship among women regarding childbearing and children. I think of the many times I've heard the horrors of pregnancy and delivery from one woman, just to hear another in her company trump her with something even worse. I always wait until everyone is finished singing the woes of delivering an eight-pound infant until I chime in with my one-ounce-under-eleven-pounder. These are the feminine equivalents of war stories, and in some cases, fish stories. The accounts of our sufferings serve as our medals of honor. The more difficult our circumstances, the greater our claim to maternal glory.

Exaggerating our sacrifices and minimizing our blessings, however, produces only exasperation in our hearts. Focusing on the difficulties we face during the long haul, we allow them to overshadow and sour us. Self-centeredness easily spills into our relationships with our children. We say we love our children, but we also try every means available to get out from under them. We can't wait until that baby is born, or until he's in bed for the night, or until school begins again. Under the yoke of what we must bear, we are tempted to view not only the struggles of pregnancy, but pregnancy itself — and even our children — as burdensome.

Mary didn't have it any easier than the vast majority of us. As exciting as it was to be the mother of the Messiah, the reality was far from fairy-tale glamour. It involved all the hardships of ordinary life. I think, if she had wished, Mary could have told many "war stories" of the struggles she faced. Yet strangely, the scriptures do not contain the agonies of Mary's trials. Rather, they record the glory of God's blessings.

The awesome responsibility given to Mary as the mother of Jesus taught her to rely on God for strength. As weak as she found herself to be, she knew that God was strong. As heavy as the burden became, she knew that she could count on him to carry her through it. Each new obstacle became a new way for God to show her how much he loved her. Although the difficulties she faced were very real, Mary knew that the glory of God was just as real — perhaps more real, because it would endure forever. Her soul was able to proclaim the greatness of God because her spirit found joy in God himself.

Just as many of us lose our sense of joy and wonder in childbearing, we often do the same in our lives of faith. We may start with a fire of love and exuberance. But as the years pass, we are sometimes lucky to end up with even a spark. We are inundated by drudgery of the spirit. We spend so much of our time counting the cost of discipleship, that we forget who paid the bill in the first place. We make so much of our own sacrifices, that we lose sight of the one who sacrificed everything for us. We talk a great deal about our "crosses", but not much about his. Faith becomes burdensome to us.

We often act as if it is Christ who demands that we carry heavy loads. We plod along, bowing low under the weight of faithfulness. But surely, this joyless existence is not what discipleship is meant to be. Indeed, life can be heavy and burdensome. But the giver of life and eternal life does not abandon us to our own weakness. The scriptures teach us that his "power is made perfect in weakness" (2 Corinthians 12:9) and that "the joy of the Lord is [our] strength" (Nehemiah 8:10).

When life weighs us down Jesus invites us to come to him. He promises to refresh our souls. Even though in the cross he carries the weight of the sins of the world, he tells us that his yoke is easy. It is because in comparison to the joy of salvation, the pains he endured, though great, were as nothing.

Light is the burden that Jesus offers us. If, like Mary, we took his yoke upon ourselves and learned from him, we would see his presence in our lives as the pure gift of grace. There is no greater thrill. If we would cultivate hearts like his — full of meekness and humility — perhaps we also would call our burdens light.

O Lord, when I first heard your call it rang like music in my ears. When I first began to walk with you, my steps were quick and sure. My heart blossomed with new-found love. My spirit was giddy with joy.

But somewhere along the way, Lord, I grew cold. The sound of your voice became too familiar. My feet began to ache from the long and difficult road. My heart became preoccupied, and my soul weighed down.

Restore to me, O God, the sweetness of that first taste of you. Rekindle in me a new fire of devotion, and reawaken in me a passion for your presence. Teach me the love that bears all things, that makes all things new, that calls all burdens light. And give me a meek and humble heart, that I might find strength in your joy.

Amen.

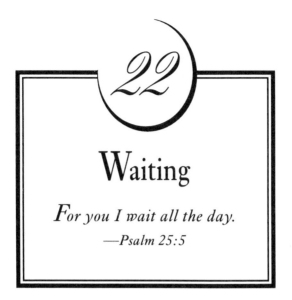

Waiting

For you I wait all the day.
—*Psalm 25:5*

As I get older, I have come to the conclusion that time flies whether you're having fun or not. It seems that each year passes more quickly than the last; that Christmas comes on the heels of the Fourth of July; and that children grow far too fast for their own good. Life roars past at such a pace that we hardly have time to catch our breath.

Pregnancy, however, has a clock all its own. It's puzzling how in some cases forty weeks can seem like forty days, and in others like forty years. Acquaintances always appear to have children in record time, while friends and relatives move steadily along course. But what I could never understand is why everyone else's pregnancies are over quickly, while mine seem to go on forever!

Certainly, in the great scheme of things, nine months is a drop in the bucket of eternity. Nonetheless, while we are pregnant, nine months can feel a lot like eternity. After the initial excitement wears off, the whole thing begins to resemble the forty years of wandering in the desert. We have the sense that we are going nowhere fast, or just wasting time walking in circles. Our frustration makes it easy to doubt whether or not a promised land even exists.

Other people often contribute to our growing impatience with their own. I remember my older girls constantly flipping the kitchen calendar back and forth, counting the weeks until the due date. Most of our conversation circled around the new baby, and whether I thought he would be early or late. My husband the computer expert was always prepared to calculate the number of hours until the projected birth. The whole thing was much like a vacation in the family car. Everything seemed to echo with incessant "are-we-there-yets?"

Waiting is never easy. When there's something to look forward to, or something we wish would end, we say "I just can't wait." Yet, for most of us, a great deal of our lives is spent waiting. Whether we can or not, is immaterial. Waiting is something we all must do. It is the emotional and spiritual equivalent of death and taxes.

In our "ten items or less" world of instant gratification, we have lost the ability to wait well. Rather than embrace the natural rhythms of life, I think many of us have sought to make our lives a continual feast. Most of us have abolished fasting of any kind. We have considered such things arcane, unnecessary, and undesirable. Because we no longer see the value of doing without, we refuse hunger. But in so doing, we also refuse what hunger can teach us. We diminish not only the purpose, but the joy of the feast.

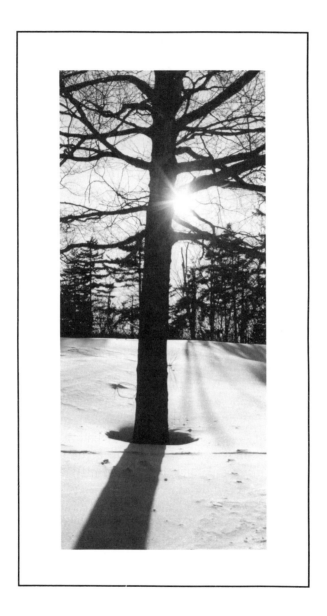

We act more like gluttonous consumers than grateful stewards.

For me, the long weeks of pregnancy is the fast before the feast, the Lenten desert before the Easter of new life. As aggravating as waiting is, it sets the stage for the great joy that accompanies birth. The longing, wonder, and anticipation that dominates — and irritates — us, is what makes childbearing satisfying. It is the emptiness that makes us full, and the thirst which allows us to be quenched.

When I think of Mary waiting for the birth of her son, I see the whole world waiting silently and unknowingly with her. The aspirations and longings of all human history are contained in those short forty weeks of her life. For, from the beginning, people of every nation have sought the divine presence. After Christ himself, the expectant Virgin Mary is both the crown and summation of all humanity. She is the expression of all souls hungering for their creator; awaiting his promised redemption. It was not for a mere nine months that the world awaited the birth of Christ, but for all time.

In my own life, I have found it much easier to wait for a new baby than to wait for God. At least we know that all pregnancies do, in fact, come to an end. But sometimes, in our spiritual lives, there seems to be no end to the waiting we must endure. Many of us become very impatient with God. We grumble like the children of Israel in the desert. We would rather he keep his miracles to himself, and bring us to the fullness of the promise without delay.

We often persist in the fear that when we need God, he will not come. Or, that if he does, it will be too late. But the fullness of the promise only comes in the fullness of time. Our God, whether we like it or not, is the Lord of the eleventh hour, fifty-ninth minute, and fifty-ninth second. He seems to live "in the nick of time"; and in the hesitation of our voices as we struggle to say, "Jesus, I trust in you."

The irony of pregnancy is that all our impatience comes from waiting for someone who is not only already with us, but actually within us. Similarly, the mystery of our faith is that we await the coming of a God who is already here and always near to us. He never loses patience with us; nor does the fire of his passion for us die down. God is always coming to us, but we are not always able to receive him.

Waiting in faith is more than spiritual thumb-twiddling. It is the fuel for the hope and desire which burns in our souls. Waiting centers our attention on whatever it is we are waiting for. We need to wait, because although God is always focused on us, we seldom fix ourselves on him. God gives us time to ripen our hearts. He knows that every apple picked too soon will be sour.

The time to ripen can seem to last forever. Many of us feel as if we have waited a lifetime for God to answer a prayer, or make himself known to us. It is like waiting to hear the final note of a symphony; or watching a football game in which the last two minutes of play last half an hour. We grow exasperated waiting for our turn in line. Our faith burns down like candles on a Advent wreath lit week after week. Sometimes in struggling to keep the vigil, we lose hope that God will ever have time for us.

Beyond time, however, there is someone else who waits. From all eternity, God has waited for each one of us to turn to him. For all eternity, he waits for us to embrace him with our whole hearts. He who was, who is, and who is to come, has already come to us. Yet, until we come to him, God's

Advent never ends — and Christmas comes only in the hearts of those who attend to his presence.

━━━━━━━━━━━━━━━━━

O Lord, you pursue my soul like a passionate lover. You are always at my heels, not even a step behind me. You are close enough to hear the whispers of my heart. You have fixed your attentions on me forever.

Yet when I turn to reach for you, you seem to vanish, Lord. You become a master of hesitation and delay. Your voice is silent, your touch is withdrawn. My soul searches for you and does not find you. I wait impatiently for you to come, and wonder if you will ever arrive.

Lord, remind me that it is not I — but you — who wait. Teach me to trust in you, and to wait well. Center my whole being on you, O God. And help me to live in this day, but not for it. Rather set my heart on what is eternal, and ripen my soul for your harvest.

Amen.

━━━━━━━━━━━━━━━━━

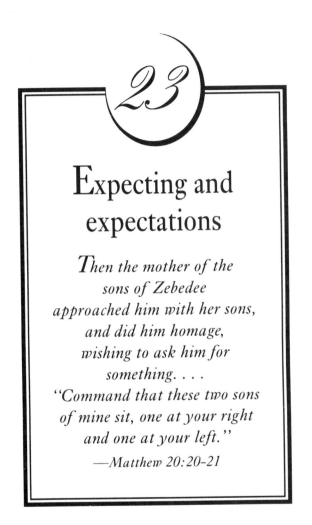

Expecting and expectations

Then the mother of the sons of Zebedee approached him with her sons, and did him homage, wishing to ask him for something. . . .
"Command that these two sons of mine sit, one at your right and one at your left."
—*Matthew 20:20–21*

Music has always been an important part of my life. Naturally, I planned on sharing it with my children. Although I had studied several musical instruments, I had always wanted to try the harp. When I found myself expecting our first child, I thought about how wonderful it would be if that child could learn to play the harp. In fact, I did a lot more than think about it. I bought several recordings of harp music, and systematically played at least one of them every day. I even "piped them in" by occasionally putting headphones on my stomach! Thankfully, I had no time to pursue such foolishness with our second child.

When our girls got older, I asked them to think carefully about which instrument they might like to play. If it suited their ability, and our budget, we would go with it. Without any hesitation, our second daughter came up with the flute. And to my delight, our oldest daughter said the harp!

I couldn't believe it had actually worked! Sadly, however, we quickly discovered that the harp was far too expensive. The instrument itself could be rented, but the instruction alone was three times more than it was for other instruments. Moreover, instructors were few and far between, and most of them were not interested in teaching a seven year old. The harp was simply not in the cards — even though I had stacked the deck. Instead, our oldest girl has pursued ballet with a passion, and our second daughter has indeed begun to play the flute.

All mothers have hopes both for themselves and for their children. But if we allow these hopes to become expectations, we will be very disappointed. We all hope to leave the hospital maternity ward in our pre-pregnancy clothes. (I even packed mine my first two times through.) Similarly, we have definite ideas of how our babies will develop: sit by six months, crawl by nine, walk by twelve. But these ideas can entrap us. Many a mother has sheepishly apologized for children who don't "measure up" in

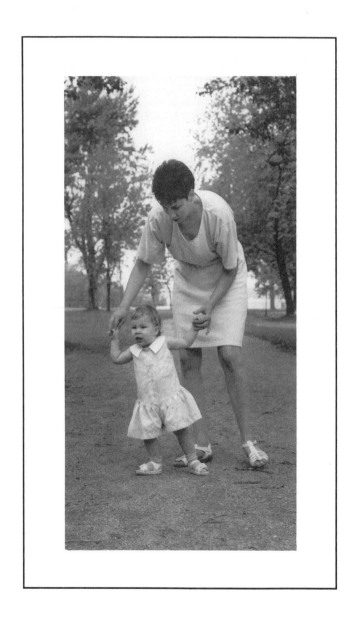

these often arbitrary ways. I know how embarrassed I was with our son, who refused to say anything intelligible until he was nearly three.

Beyond those early milestones our expectations change, but they do not disappear. The potty soon gives way to ABC's, math facts, and report cards; and climbing the stairs is replaced by little league and dance recitals. Eventually, all the things of childhood evolve into concerns about colleges, jobs, marriages, and grandchildren.

However it is we choose to define "perfect," most of us want "perfect" children. There is no such thing as an impartial parent. We all believe that our kids are the best. But there are times that some of us cross into demanding that they be so.

In the process of doing all we can for our kids, the line between the hopes we have had for ourselves and those we have for our children can become blurred. In loving our children, we want them to succeed. We want to keep them from making our mistakes. We hope that they will do more than we did, and become more than we are. But some of us end up looking to them to fulfill some of the dreams we have laid aside for ourselves. Somewhere along the line we stop giving ourselves to our children freely. Instead, we begin investing ourselves in them, expecting some kind of return.

Our agendas inevitably interfere with the unconditional love our children need. Regardless of what they are, our expectations orient our children toward ourselves. They often serve more as obstacles to our approval than as tools of personal development. Moreover, they elevate the importance of our approval, often at the expense of God's glory. If I had pushed even harder, my daughter may indeed have become a harpist. But at what cost? What desires of hers, and more importantly, what divine purpose would have been squelched in the process?

When Mary took her part in God's plan for salvation, she gave up not only the expectations she had for herself, but also those for the divine child she would bear. No doubt, as the mother of Jesus, Mary possessed tremendous influence. Nonetheless, she did not push her own agenda on either her son, or on God. She made herself the handmaid of the Lord. She did not seek to define or influence his purpose. She only sought to serve it. Mary knew that not only was her son perfect, but so was the plan God would bring to fulfillment in him.

Whatever her ideas would have been, Mary surrendered them to the purpose God had in mind. Rather than having hopes for her son, she chose to place her hopes in him. The truth is that, like most of us, Mary did not know what to expect — only whom. She could not anticipate the events of her life, either good or bad. She did not know what time would reveal. Expecting Jesus, Mary expected salvation and nothing else. She held on to the promise, and let go of everything else.

Letting go, however, does not mean distancing ourselves from our children. Rather, it is surrendering our claims of ownership over them. I think that Joseph is the clearest example of letting go without drawing back. Without a doubt Mary's baby threw a wrench in the works of just about all of Joseph's expectations. Engaged to a virgin, Joseph suddenly found himself in strange and deep waters.

But instead of turning his back on Mary and her child, Joseph drew nearer to them both. For their sake, he embraced the unknown and mysterious will of God, and accepted the difficult ways of God. In that moment, Joseph not only welcomed God's child as his own, but in place of children that would have been his own. Rather than sulking over unfulfilled expectations, Joseph responded in faith. He risked believing that God would give him more, and not less. In the end, he was not disappointed.

Mary and Joseph teach us that the need to let go of our expectations begins even before our babies are born. In all reality, our children are not only ours. They belong, as we all do, to God. It is he who entrusts them to our care.

But God not only trusts us with the care of our children's needs; he gives us their potential as well. As parents, we are responsible for developing fully our children's abilities. For while our children are children, God leaves in our hands the purpose he embeds in every person he creates. The excellence of our parenting is perhaps best measured by how much our children progress in accomplishing God's plans — not ours and not theirs — for their lives. We instruct them best by following his will ourselves.

As disciples of Jesus, each of us is entrusted with the spiritual potential we possess in faith. Most of us spend lots of time trying to discern what our gifts are, and how to develop them. Unfortunately, many of us retreat into labels of faith. We characterize ourselves as "traditional" or "charismatic," "active" or "contemplative." But in defining ourselves in these ways, we box our souls into a lifetime of predetermined spiritual practice.

Allowing wherever we are at any point in time to evolve into spiritual expectations interferes with God's ability to lead us deeper. When we narrow the spectrum of how we will allow God to move in us, we anticipate more, and participate less. We train our spirits to expect things from God, rather than God himself. And when we don't get what we expect, we are disappointed.

But if we allowed God's hopes to take precedence over our own expectations, we would never be disappointed. His hopes for us are far beyond what we could hope for ourselves. If we could learn to distance ourselves from ourselves, we would draw closer to him. He tells us that if we would only seek his kingdom first, we would have everything else besides (Matthew 6:33). How much happier we would be, if letting go of everything else, we would learn to cling to God alone.

O Lord, with you all things are possible! You walk on water, you heal the sick, you even raise the dead. You give hope to the distressed, no one who hopes in you is disappointed.

But Lord, I have been disappointed in you. For there are many times when you are slow to answer me; when you lead me down paths that I don't want to take, times when my dreams lie shattered around me.

Deliver me, O God, from expecting things, and teach me to expect you alone. Keep me from plans and ideas that are mine, but not yours. Help me to embrace your hopes as my own. Give me a faith that surrenders my claims to anything but you. Remind me that I am your servant, and not your advisor. And make me a handmaid of your perfect will.

Amen.

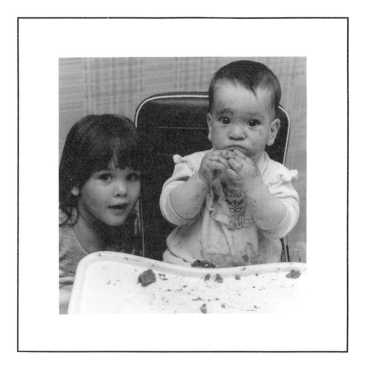

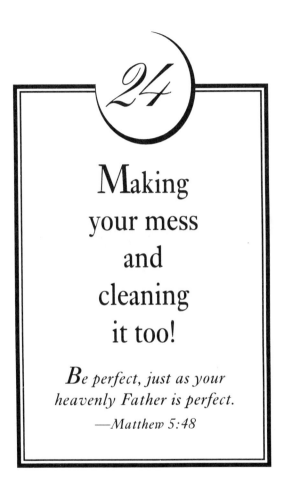

Making your mess and cleaning it too!

Be perfect, just as your heavenly Father is perfect.
—*Matthew 5:48*

Before I had children, I didn't think much about how to raise them. But when we began having a family, it seemed as if we could think of little else. I remember having plenty of discussion with my husband about parenting, especially regarding discipline. But in those early years of inexperience, it was all by trial and error — and believe me, it was more error than anything else.

As much as I wanted perfect children, I wanted even more to be a perfect mother. I remember the terror I felt during that first drive home from the hospital. I wondered, what in the world was I supposed to do with this thing? Was it really all just a question of following natural maternal instincts? There were countless stories of mothers who had scarred their children for life. Obviously, they had done something wrong. But I wasn't sure how to avoid it, because I couldn't be sure what it was. I supposed you could judge the tree by it's fruit. Obviously "bad" mothers produced "bad" children. But there were too many examples to the contrary. And if you waited that long to find out if what you were doing was right, it would be too late.

To me, the greatest challenge of child raising was, and is, discipline. Being a hot-tempered person with high standards for children's behavior, I often lost patience with my young children. Sometimes my expectations of them were off the mark. Other times, my ideas of how best to deal with a situation got me into a bind. I remember one incident in particular with our second very strong-willed daughter. I had already warned, yelled, smacked, and sent her to her room. I had no alternatives left. Still defiant, I threatened to throw her out the window. I almost meant it.

Not knowing where to turn, I concluded that perhaps the best way to learn how to be a good mother was to watch other women doing it. I saw parents who were more strict, and those who were more lenient; those who were highly interventionist, and those who were rather laissez-faire. I observed many women talking calmly to their misbehaving children, never raising their voices, and never ever spanking them. In contrast, I remembered in my own upbringing a good deal of hollering, and a few smacks when I was particularly disobedient. The whole thing was inconclusive, as the results were very mixed.

Next I tried the textbook approach. At the suggestion of some friends who were at a loss themselves, I resorted to some of the methods and techniques suggested by parenting "experts." I remember debating which chair I would designate as the "time-out chair," and getting together the various materials I would need as if I were setting up a laboratory. The one thing I never did figure out was which one of us was the guinea pig!

Invariably, every book stressed the importance of consistency with children. That turned out to be my downfall with all of them. As hard as I tried, I could not maintain consistency in any of these methods. I just couldn't keep up the front of acting like someone I wasn't twenty-four hours a day. Frustrated and exhausted, I threw up my hands, and rolled up my sleeves.

It finally occurred to me that as much as my own weaknesses got in the way of being a good mother, trying to eliminate them made things even worse. The fact was that I was the mother of my children. To be sure, I had my share of faults and limitations, but so did my children. So did everybody. The quality of my mothering was not dependent on how many books I had read, or which expert advice I followed. It depended on what kind of a person I was. Things got better when I recognized that despite all the advice I could gather, and regardless of how hard I tried, I was going to make mistakes as a mother. Both my children and I would suffer the consequences of those mistakes. But we could also learn from them.

As the mother of Jesus, Mary must have been continually aware of her limitations. She was, after all, a young and inexperienced mother. I'm sure, too, that Mary had her share of challenges in raising her son. She must have felt the weight of the enormous responsibility she had. If she failed as a mother, there was no telling what dreadful consequences could follow.

There were no Dr. Spocks in ancient Israel. The only expert advice Mary would have would come from the women in her village, and any guidance her mother might give. And when circumstances forced the Holy Family to depart for Egypt, she left all of them behind. In a land of strangers, like the rest of us, Mary had to find her own way.

Mary was well aware of the importance of her task, and she knew her limitations as well. But Mary did not live out her life's mission in fear and anxiety. Rather, she approached her work as she did God, with confidence— that is with faith. Mary knew that there was no mask to hide behind that God could not see through. She didn't try to be someone better, someone wiser, or someone stronger than she was. It was not because she believed in herself, but because she believed in God. Whether or not there was someone better, or wiser, or stronger for the job, he had chosen her.

There are times for all of us when we are certain only of our own inadequacies, and afraid of what others may think. In those times, many of us resort to masking who we really are. Not even realizing what we are doing, we hide behind pretense to protect ourselves from failure. We act out our lives rather than live them. Like important papers hidden in a special place for safe keeping, we put our true selves away. But when we need them, we forget where it was we put them.

As hard as it is to be someone other than who we are in the presence of others, it is even harder to do it in the presence of the God who made us. Nonetheless, many of us attempt to do exactly that. Afraid to be our poor selves with him, we put on all the "holy" things we think God wants of us. We come to him with all the perfection we can muster. We even design elaborate methods to reach him. But the truth is that the life of faith must be mothered, not engineered. There are no high-tech highways to heaven.

God has no use for our spiritual techniques or fig leaves. He does not want us to hide ourselves in false piety and feigned holiness; and he's not impressed with our staged performances. What pleases God is faith, pure and simple. Not faith in our strength and holiness, but in his loving mercy toward our weakness, and sin. In this faith God gives us hope, that someday "we shall be like him, for we shall see him as he is" (1 John 3:2).

O Lord, you are a holy God. You are perfect wisdom, gentle strength, and unbridled love. What is there in me for you to desire? Yet, you created me in your image to reflect your glory.

Lord, how can I come to you as I am? For your shallows are too deep for me. Before your gentleness I am weak. And by the light of your love I see the poverty of my own.

Help me to approach you without fear, O God. Strip away any pretense or falsity from my soul. Center my faith in your mercy, Lord, and not in my own works or worth. Teach me to accept those you choose, even when they are not my choice. For now, Lord, hide me beneath your wings. But one day, show me your face and make me like yourself.

Amen.

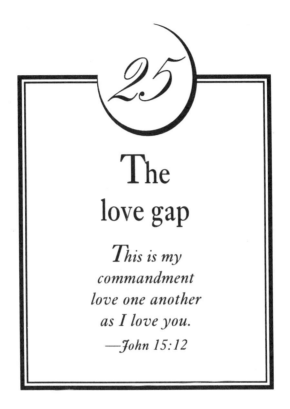

25

The love gap

This is my commandment love one another as I love you.
—John 15:12

A day or two after our first child was born, I sat down in my hospital room to make a list of the things the baby would need. I already had all the big items, but in no time at all the paper was filled. Diapers, undershirts, sleepers, socks, baby powder, pacifiers, shampoo, hooded towels, receiving blankets — the list went on and on.

As I was dressing our new baby to leave the hospital, the pediatrician came in for a last check-up. She asked if I had everything ready at home. But when I showed her my list, she said something I will never forget. "All she needs is warmth." I knew she was right. All my baby would ever need was warmth. What I didn't know, was whether I could give it to her.

I quickly found that the biggest obstacle to that warmth wasn't time or money, it was my selfishness. There is nothing better than a new baby to show us just how self-centered we are. I know how many times I've rolled over when my children have woken up at night, or made them wait just because I was busy doing something for myself. To a greater or lesser degree, we all live for ourselves. Love, however, teaches us to live for others. The warmth our children need comes from that love — the kind that asks us not only to put our wants on the back burner, but to take them entirely off the stove.

Children bring about great changes in our lives. After kids, we no longer eat the same, sleep the same, do the same things, or even like the same things we did B.C. — before children. It's not that we suddenly fall in love with big canaries or purple dinosaurs. But in loving our children, we direct more of our lives toward them, and less toward ourselves. We begin to move beyond ourselves from selfishness to love.

When love conquers selfishness, it propels us in directions we would not otherwise choose. Certainly, nobody wants to change diapers, or get up for a night feeding. Nevertheless, we all do these things for our children because we love them. We may not like sports much, or opera either. But if we have a child with a great pitch or perfect pitch, chances are nothing will keep us out of the ballpark or the theater. Indeed, most of us love our children more than life itself. We do everything in our power

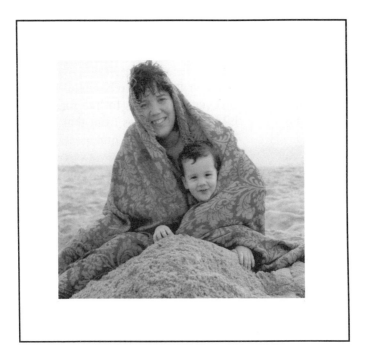

to fill all their needs and many of their desires. We cover them with all the warmth and love we can muster.

But no matter how much we love our children, we cannot be there for them all the time, and we cannot give them everything they want or need. None of us are able to protect our children from the consequences of their own choices, let alone from the choices others make. The world can be a cold, cold place. At times, the warmth we can give them is as insufficient as an umbrella in a hurricane.

Deep inside we all know that our love alone is simply not enough. There will always be a gap between the love each of us needs and what we can receive, even from the most loving of parents, spouses, or children. This "love gap" exists for every man, woman, and child. It is rooted in the love-hunger of our souls, which far surpasses what any human being could give us. Try as we may to fill the gap, we will never succeed in doing so.

The fact is that although parents stand in the place of God, none of us is God. Our shortcomings, however, don't just amount to our inability to perform miracles, or command the wind and the waves. What makes us lacking is not our inability to do what God does, but our inability to love as God loves.

Throughout the life of Jesus, Mary's love for him is clear. She attends to his needs. She supports him in ministry. She never abandons him, even when nearly all his disciples did. Though powerless, she stands lovingly beneath the cross.

Nevertheless, while Mary gave everything she was to her son, she never made the mistake of thinking that her love would be enough. She knew her human limitations — that she alone was insufficient. She knew, too, that without anything or anyone else, God alone would suffice. Mary had seen him to be all-knowing and all-powerful. And more than that, she had come to understand that God's knowledge and power did not reside in his mind or in his might, but in his perfect love.

Mary knew that however much we love our children, God loves them — and us — even more. This was her source of peace as she set about raising her son. There would be gaps in her motherly love for Jesus. But God would fill them, just as he had for her — not sparingly, but to overflowing.

It is humbling to realize that as much as our children need us, they need God even more. As our children grow into adulthood, in some sense, they need us less and less. But as they assume the responsibilities and challenges of adult life, they will need God more and more. Although without us our children will die, without God, they will never live.

The weakness of human love will fail us. Yet it is comforting to know that divine love never fails. Instead of scorning our weaknesses, God chooses to perfect his strength in them. Rather than giving us just enough of his love to get by meagerly, God floods our souls with his passion. He loves us without limits of any kind. God never ceases to love, for love is not merely his occupation. It is his identity — "God is love" (1 John 4:8).

When we come to grips with our many failures to love, we need only to turn to the love who lives in our hearts. Instead of struggling to love on our own power, we need to allow ourselves to be overpowered by the love of the Holy Trinity. We must fan the fires of the divine passion that burns for us and in us with our lives. Likewise, we must teach our children to turn to God.

God has not left us without the means to secure for our children the love they need. Knowing the shallowness of our human love, God has provided us all with a deeper well from which to draw. It is possible to assure that our children will receive all the love they need for the rest of their lives. But to do so, we must give them more than ourselves. We must give them Christ. All the canyons of our inadequacies, however immense, can be bridged; but only by the grace which flows from his outstretched arms.

O God, by the power of perfect love, you called each of us into existence. You created us to walk in love with one another and with you. You shaped our souls to be the channels through which your love would flood the world.

Yet so often, Lord, I dam up your love with selfishness. Sometimes only a few drops can be squeezed from my heart. In truth I don't love anyone as much I as I love myself — let alone as you have loved me.

Lord, I have believed and I have worked, teach me now to love. Help me to give myself to you, so that I may give you to those around me. Lord, move my heart from selfishness to love, and live in my soul as the God who is love itself.

Amen.

26

Labor and delivery: birthing Christ in our lives

*When a woman is in labor
she is in anguish
because her hour has arrived;
but when she has given birth
to a child, she remembers the pain
no longer, because of her joy
that a child has been born
into the world.*

—John 16:21

The purpose of pregnancy is birth. But whenever I find out I'm pregnant, my first thought is that I don't want to go through labor. Like everyone else, I took the Lamaze class the first time through. When my turn came, however, I discovered that there really isn't much that anyone can do to prepare for childbirth.

There is a certain charm to the naiveté we all have about labor and delivery before we've been there ourselves. In my case, that blissful ignorance is captured on film. The first photograph in our oldest daughter's baby album is one of me standing at the door of our apartment with suitcase in hand. My hair is in place, my makeup is done, and I'm smiling broadly. It was taken just before I left for the hospital.

Needless to say, that smile didn't last any longer than the hair and makeup. My innocence regarding birth fell rather quickly to the wayside. But when I happen across that photo now I can't help but think of it as the last glimpse of the much younger, very inexperienced me. I smile to think of how I was then — and cry a little too.

The reality of childbirth is a far cry from what most of us imagine it to be. As a child I remember thinking that a dotted line would appear on a woman's belly, and a trap door would open to let the baby out. I have to admit that some of my adult ideas weren't much more accurate.

My husband had his own set of misconceptions. To me, it seemed as though he was trying out for Lamaze labor coach of the year. He was ready to assume ice-chip and breathing patrol from the moment we were wheeled into the labor room. After a few hours of "pant, pant, blow," he became so annoying that I actually punched him in the

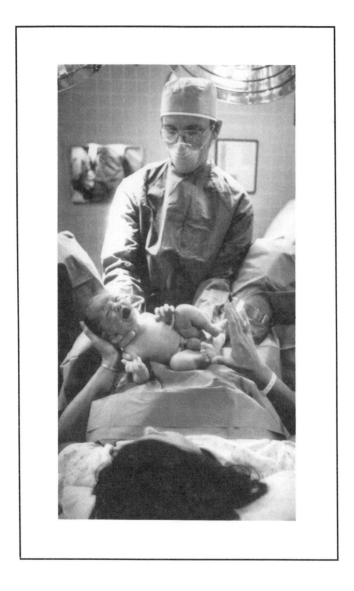

stomach! In the three births that followed, my husband learned to stay in the corner and keep his head low.

In addition to our own notions, there are all kinds of wisdom regarding childbirth to be found. Historically, "feminine folklore" offered advice which was sometimes rather bizarre. My grandmother, for example, heard that if you fall asleep during labor, you were condemned to walk around with your eyes half-closed for the rest of your life. The attending nurse during her first birth must have thought my grandmother was crazy when she asked if it was alright to sleep through labor.

Today such a tale would meet with immediate laughter. In our modern sophistication we have indeed traded mythology for a much more scientific approach to birth. From my perspective, however, a thorough knowledge of centimeters doesn't do any more for a woman in the delivery room than old rumors did.

There's no getting around the fact that having a baby hurts. Whether you have an "easy" birth or a difficult one, the pain of labor and delivery puts us all at the very edge of existence. Childbirth, like no other experience, unites our physical, emotional, and spiritual selves at the limits of who and what we are. The intensity of sense and emotion, and the enormous significance of the birth event, both focuses and overwhelms us. Once labor has begun, there's no turning back. We're in for the duration whether we like it or not. We are all at once the happiest and the most miserable we have ever been.

Although we all gain as much support and encouragement as we can, when the time comes, only a mother can birth her child. Isolated by the pain and the total involvement birth demands, each of us is in a real sense alone.

Nurses, doctors, and fathers may all be in attendance, but none of them can do much more than wait and watch. As my great-grandmother used to say: "The Queen of England has servants to do everything for her. But when it comes to having a baby, even she has to do it herself."

Mary, too, did it herself. Young and inexperienced, without her mother, and far from home, Mary brought Jesus into the world. There were no classes to prepare her, nor was there any scientific explanation for her to hear. All she had at her disposal was her inner strength. If anyone deserved a "birthing room" equipped with whirlpool, television, and the best of medical care, it was Mary. But for her and the Son of God, a dark and dirty stable sufficed. There was no anesthesiologist standing by. Only her love for God and his son would see her through it.

Romanticized Christmas images aside, the birth of Christ is an accurate picture of the new birth God offers each of us. Like all babies, his birth was accomplished by pain and hard work, and accompanied by water and blood. Eternal life is much the same. Salvation was birthed in the pain of the cross. When Jesus' side was pierced by a lance, water and blood flowed forth. We come to that moment of new birth ourselves in the sacramental waters of baptism and the eucharistic blood of Christ.

We all know that it is impossible to give birth without labor. Yet, when it comes to birthing the new life of the spirit, suddenly we expect something else. Many of us shrink from the hard work of faith. Some of us struggle to stay pregnant rather than go through what it takes to give birth to a new life of the soul. All of us resist the pain and anguish that often accompanies spiritual growth.

Just as pregnancy is for the purpose of birthing a child, faith is for the purpose of birthing Christ. No one would become pregnant as an end in itself; and yet, many of us tend to view faith in that very way. What we need to understand is that Mary's call to bring forth Christ into the world is not unlike our own. Jesus first dwelt in Mary's womb, so that he could enter the world through her. Likewise, he dwells in our hearts by grace so that he may continually enter the world through us.

Filled with his Spirit, our souls are nurtured, and grow, and wait. Finally, the tiny seed of divine presence that once began silent and unnoticed, grows beyond our ability to carry it any longer. The Christ within us becomes strong enough to be exposed to the world. In that hour called the fullness of time, we bring him forth, through our hearts and into our world. Our lives become the birthplace of Christ.

The pain of growing in faith is the pain of birth. If we suffer great pains in delivering a child, can we expect to suffer nothing in birthing Christ? Our hearts are no larger than our wombs. But despite the pain of labor and delivery, no one doubts whether a child is worth it. Similarly, no disciple of Jesus, even those who suffered martyrdom, would regret their willingness to accept the cross. The joy of his intimate presence far outweighs any pain suffered to attain it.

How simple it is, Lord, to embark on the journey, to begin the struggle, to enter the fray. And how difficult it is to finish the race, to complete the task, to endure till the end. The fantasies are quickly and easily embraced, but reality is heavy and hard to bear.

Overwhelmed by my own pain, Lord, I forget what you suffered. I resist any growth that hurts. I shrink from the pangs that bring you forth. I want all of the blessings, and none of the labor.

Lord, help me to love you even when it hurts. In the pain be my companion, and beyond it be my joy. Grow within me until I must bring you forth. Lead my heart to the fullness of time. And when my hour comes, Lord, burst forth with new life from my soul.

Amen.

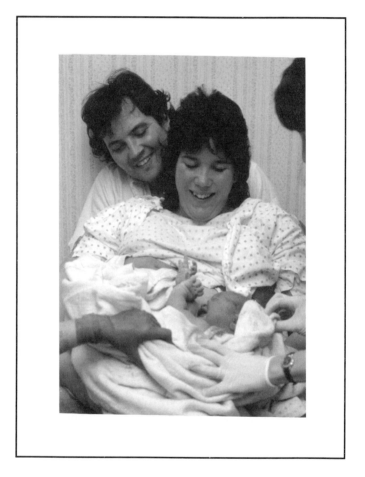

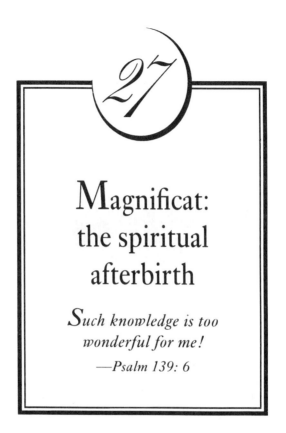

Magnificat: the spiritual afterbirth

Such knowledge is too wonderful for me!
—*Psalm 139: 6*

Although each pregnancy and delivery is unique, for me the final chapter of birth has always been the same. Tired as I was after the ordeal of giving birth, I could never seem to rest much. With each new baby's arrival, I spent the night following labor simply too excited to fall asleep. Invariably, I've found myself during those wee morning hours thanking God for the miracle of new life.

187

A new baby makes our whole family more aware of how much there is to be grateful for. Tiny fingers and toes rekindle our wonder at life, and renew our sense of its frailty. The birth experience invites us all to be thankful for one another. Our two older girls have actually thanked me for having their little brother and sister.

Pregnancy and birth is mysterious and marvelous. Indeed, the whole process from start to finish is nothing less than miraculous. When we first receive those tiny babies into our arms, it's hard to believe that we had anything at all to do with bringing them into the world. What a gift it is to be not only a spectator, but an instrument in bringing about new life. To think that just moments before, the little one we hold lived inside us, is beyond the grasp of our understanding. It just doesn't seem possible — let alone real.

To me, it seems strange that such a wonderful thing is so common to our experience. Unlike the Olympics or Haley's Comet, women give birth every day. Black and red, yellow and white, the great variety of humanity is recreated with each new day. As different as we are from one another, and as different as the lives we live are, child-bearing is the common denominator of human experience. Yet, it is inexpressibly awesome every time it happens.

But as wonderful as pregnancy is, the God who blesses us with pregnancy is even more wonderful. He is the origin of all life; and he is the ultimate destiny of all living things. God not only makes all of us, he cares for each of us. God not only gives us life, he calls us to share his divine life. God is always with us and within us. He longs for us to live with him, and in him.

In knowing this wondrous God, Mary was especially blessed. It did not take a virgin birth to convince Mary of the power of God's love towards her. She had always known it. But unlike most of us, Mary never lost her sense of awe for God; and she never took him for granted.

In her humility, Mary knew that she could never earn God's love. She could only accept it. Throughout her life, Mary's posture towards God is one of profound gratitude. It is, I think, the most attractive and compelling thing about her. I have never heard anyone shout "thank you." That is why there is nothing loud or ungentle about Mary. Her whole life was lived out in thanks to God.

In the scriptures, Mary's words are few. But knowing her spirit, it is not surprising to find that the longest passage attributed to Mary is her beautiful prayer of gratitude, the Magnificat. Like Mary's life, her words are wholly directed to God. In exuberant joy she speaks of her blessedness, not because of anything she had done, but because God had "looked upon [her] lowliness" (Luke 1:48).

Interestingly, this prayer was not offered in private. While the annunciation occurred in secret between the angel and Mary, the gratitude she voiced in the Magnificat was a public act of worship. Mary's words recall God faithfulness and his love. Proclaiming it aloud, she shares the coming of God's salvation in Christ Jesus with Elizabeth, and with us. With the words of the Magnificat, Mary leads us all in giving thanks to God.

Although we easily recognize that God worked miracles in Mary's life, we often fail to recognize that the Almighty has done great things for all of us as well. God gives us life, new life, and eternal life. Like Mary, we must learn to culti-

vate hearts that are not grudging, but grateful. It is in gratitude that the work of God becomes clear to us. Gratitude
reveals much of what is hidden by human pretense and
pride.

More than giving credit where it is due, gratefulness to
God secures our joy in difficult times. The psalmist teaches
us that "God inhabits the praises of his people." Moreover,
we "enter his gates with thanksgiving, his courts with
praise" (Psalm 100:4). If we want to live as Mary did, in the
continual presence of God, we must learn to thank and
praise him. Only then will our souls magnify the Lord, and
only then will our spirits find joy in him.

As our unborn children growing within us shape our
bodies, Christ in our hearts will shape our lives. He will
lead us through times of anticipation and excitement, as
well as times of exasperation and waiting. He will stir in us
immeasurable joy, and he will bring us to the point of complete surrender. His spirit will grow in us until we can hold
him no longer, until, in labor and in pain, Jesus bursts forth
from our hearts.

Just as our children teach us a great deal, there is much
that we learn through faith about God and ourselves.
Nevertheless, such enlightenment is not the object of faith.
While our objectives are often clouded and mixed, God's
purpose is single and clear. Everything God does origi-
nates in love, operates by love, and is directed towards
love. The great gift of faith is the love, love that flows freely
when we allow God to embrace us intimately. It is God's
will that as we allow him to embrace our hearts, we will
come to embrace him as well. He does not want to remain
a stranger.

More than wisdom or understanding, there is unspeakable joy in the loving presence of God. It is from this joy that Mary prayed the Magnificat, and found the strength to live it completely. Most of us could spend an eternity counting our blessings. But of all we have to be thankful for, the greatest is God himself.

———

My whole heart sings your greatness, O Lord, and all that I am is alive with joy. For in my nothingness your love has sought me out. Your grace has overtaken me.

How can the world not envy me? For you have done what is impossible — what people do not even dare to dream. You stand alone in glory.

Extending your hand to all who reach for you, you uphold them with gentle strength. But the proud you disperse. By their own hands they fall.

You topple the powerful, but set the weak in high places. You give to the heart that hungers, but take away from the one who fills himself.

You will not abandon anyone who serves you, for you bind yourself to your own with mercy. You guard the fruit of your word in the hearts of those who love you; in the hearts of all you have blessed.

Amen.

———

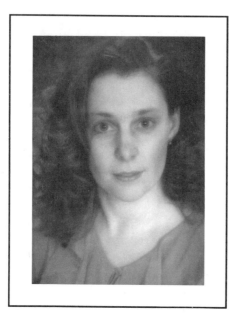

As a writer, lay evangelist, and singer-songwriter, Jaymie Stuart Wolfe seeks to use every means available to communicate the gospel. Through her *Loaves and Fishes Ministry* she performs many inspirational concerts andis a featured speaker at numerous church and spiritual gatherings. Jaymie has produced four cassettes of her original music, and her "Under My Roof" column appears regularly in *The Pilot*, Boston's Catholic newspaper. She can also be heard throughout the U.S. on Father Tom DiLorenzo's *In Season and Out of Season* radio ministry. A 1983 graduate of Harvard University and a convert to Catholicism, Jaymie is the mother of six children.